RADIONUCLIDE TREATMENTS

Edited by **Cigdem Soydal**

Radionuclide Treatments
http://dx.doi.org/10.5772/65461
Edited by Cigdem Soydal

Contributors
Elgin Ozkan, Umut Elboga, Mine Araz, Derya Cayir, Gökhan Koca, Aylin Akbulut, F. Nur Aydınbelge

Published by InTech
Janeza Trdine 9, 51000 Rijeka, Croatia

Publishing Process Manager Mirena Calmic
Technical Editor SPi Global
Cover InTech Design team

First published July, 2017
Printed in Croatia
Legal deposit, Croatia: National and University Library in Zagreb

Additional hard copies can be obtained from orders@intechopen.com

Radionuclide Treatments, Edited by Cigdem Soydal
p. cm.
Print ISBN 978-953-51-3379-7
Online ISBN 978-953-51-3380-3

For EU product safety concerns:
IN TECH d.o.o., Prolaz Marije Krucifikse Kozulić 3, 51000 Rijeka, Croatia,
info@intechopen.com or visit our website at intechopen.com.

Meet the editor

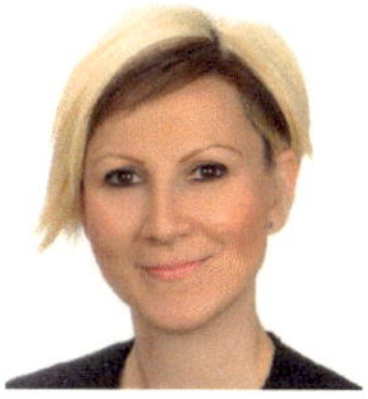

Cigdem Soydal was born in 1979 in Istanbul, Turkey. She graduated at the Medical School of Ankara University in 2004 and has been working as nuclear medicine physician at Ankara University since 2012. Her special interest areas include nuclear oncology and radionuclide treatments. She has reached the fellowship of the European Board of Nuclear Medicine degree in 2016 and has more than 50 published manuscripts in international journals and in conference books. She is a member of the Turkish Society of Nuclear Medicine and European Association of Nuclear Medicine.

Contents

Preface

In modern medicine practice, radionuclide treatments have an increasing role in the management of most benign and malignant diseases. For this reason, having baseline information on the radionuclide treatments has become mandatory for several medicine practitioners.

Radionuclide treatments have been designed as a reference book for medical oncologists, endocrinologists, and nuclear medicine physicians for initial evaluation of patients for radionuclide treatments. Pretreatment patient evaluation, administration of treatments, and posttreatment follow-up for each treatment have been included to the related chapters.

Cigdem Soydal, Editor
Ankara University,
Medical Faculty,
Department of Nuclear Medicine,
Ankara, Turkey

Section 1

Radioidoine Treatment for Benign and Malignant Thyroid Disease

Chapter 1

Radioiodine Treatment for Benign Thyroid Diseases

Aylin Akbulut, Fadimana Nur Aydinbelge and
Gökhan Koca

Additional information is available at the end of the chapter

http://dx.doi.org/10.5772/intechopen.68575

Abstract

Radioiodine (RAI) is becoming the preferred treating option for benign thyroid diseases. Hyperthyroidism is defined as hypermetabolic state caused by high levels of circulating thyroid hormones of the thyroid gland. The most common hyperthyroidism causes are Graves' disease, toxic multinodular goitre, and solitary hyperfunctioning nodule, for which RAI can be preferred as a definitive treatment option. It is rapidly incorporated into the thyroid and with its beta emissions with a path length of 1–3 mm cause extensive local tissue damage and necrosis. The thyroid gland is effectively ablated over a period of 8–18 weeks and can no more produce normal amount of thyroid hormones. It is an individualized therapy that can either be a first-line therapy, or an alternative therapy to neck surgery or to use of antithyroidal drugs after 1 year. For the optimal efficiency, before the RAI treatment, the patients should be extensively assessed and they also should be given clear information about the treatment, as well as written instructions for precautions to avoid irradiation exposure to other people. Moreover, after RAI treatment patients should have their regular follow-up. This chapter summarizes all the points for a RAI treatment.

Keywords: radioiodine treatment, hyperthyroidism, Graves' disease, toxic multinodular goitre, benign thyroid diseases

1. Introduction

Radioiodine (RAI) has been used for over 70 years as a treatment for benign thyroid diseases [1]. Regarding massive amount of past data, RAI treatment is broadly accepted as a safe and effective treatment for benign thyroid diseases with low incidence of acute or chronic adverse effects.

Thyrotoxicosis is thyroid-induced hypermetabolism, either secondary to thyroid hormone release from an overactive or inflamed thyroid gland or introduced from an extra-thyroidal

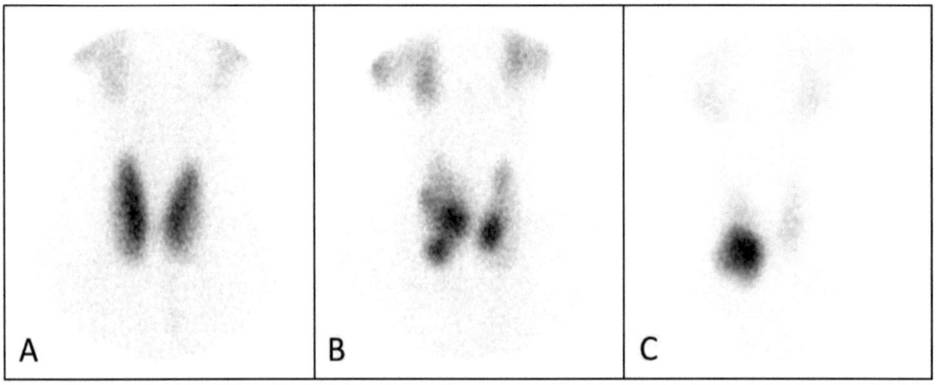

Figure 1. The thyroid scans examples of the main causes of hyperthyroidism. (A) Graves' disease, (B) toxic multinodular disease, and (C) solitary hyperfunctioning nodule.

source. A suppressed serum thyroid stimulating hormone (TSH) level, below 0.4 mU/L, confirms the diagnosis of hyperthyroidism, meaning the pathology is within the thyroid gland [2]. To differentiate the cause of hyperthyroidism, RAI uptake test can be performed and a thyroid scan can give additional information. **Figure 1** shows the thyroid scans of the main causes of hyperthyroidism: Graves' disease and toxic multinodular disease and solitary hyperfunctioning nodules.

The symptoms of hyperthyroidism are nonspecific such as tachycardia, tremor, nervousness, anxiety, heat intolerance, sweating, and weight loss.

Hyperthyroidism can be treated with antithyroid drugs (ATDs), RAI therapy, and surgery. The actual therapy selected varies on the characteristics of the patient and the underlying cause of hyperthyroidism.

The aim of RAI therapy in patients with hyperthyroidism is to achieve a nonhyperthyroidal status that is not responding to ATDs and also to reduce the size of the nodules and to decrease the symptoms related to hyperthyroidism and gland enlargement in patients with toxic nodular goiter.

This chapter includes RAI treatment for benign thyroid diseases, I131 information, administration, effect mechanism, indications and contraindications, patient preparation, I131 dose selection and withdrawal of antithyroid drugs, lithium and recombinant human TSH usage under a seperate topic, named special conditions, precautions, advers effects and patient follow-up.

2. Iodine131

I131, known as sodium iodine, is the most commonly used radionuclide therapy and also the first radiopharmaceutical to be used for the treatment of the thyroid gland in benign thyroid diseases since the 1940s [1].

The principle mechanism of RAI treatment depends on the destructive effect of the radioactivity that is directed to the target tissue thorough "cross fire effect" in a continuous manner. RAI is a beta-emitting radionuclide with a physical half-life of 8.02 days, a principal gamma ray of 364 keV, and a principal beta particle with a maximum energy of 0.61 MeV, average energy of 0.192 MeV, and average range in the tissue of 0.4 mm. The principal gamma ray of 364 keV enables imaging with a gamma camera.

Oral capsule or in liquid form is the most common way to administer to patients; however, it can also be administered intravenously. When it is swallowed, it is absorbed in the gastrointestinal tract from blood circulation and then it accumulates in the thyroid gland.

2.1. The effect mechanism

The sodium iodide symporter (NIS) is an intrinsic plasma membrane glycoprotein that mediates the active transport of iodide in the thyroid gland and also in some extrathyroidal tissues, like lactating breast, gastric mucosa, and salivary and lacrimal glands [3]. RAI uptake occurs across the basolateral membrane of thyroid follicular cells via an active transport process mediated by the NIS, like inorganic iodine.

NIS protein expression is revealed to be heterogeneous at the basolateral membrane of a minority of follicular cells in normal thyroid gland tissue [4]; it is increased in thyroid tissue in acute Graves' disease, consistent with the clinical observation of diffusely increased radioiodine uptake [5]. In toxic multinodular goiters (TMNG), heterogeneous NIS protein expression appears to be stronger than the normal thyroid gland and less than the Graves' thyroid tissue [6].

RAI is rapidly concentrated by the follicular cells and accumulated in colloid cells after iodide organification. Beta particles emitted by RAI destroy the functioning thyroid tissue. Hence, cell function is inhibited and proliferation capacity is affected by destructing follicular thyroid cell. The severity of this effect is directly proportional to the given dose.

The main effect of RAI treatment causes an intense radiation thyroiditis that leads to apoptosis and necrosis of hyperactive/active follicular thyroid cells, glandular atrophy, and loss of the thyroid capacity to synthesize and decrease thyroid hormones [7].

3. Indications and contraindications

Mainly, RAI therapy indications in benign thyroid diseases include Graves' disease, toxic multinodular goitre, solitary hyperfunctioning nodule, nontoxic multinodular goitre, goitre recurrence after surgery, and also amiodarone-induced hyperthyroidism with special precautions and ablation of residual thyroid tissue in case of malignant ophthalmopathy after surgery, but during an inactive state of the orbitopathy.

RAI therapy's absolute contraindications are pregnancy and breastfeeding, and relative contraindications are incapable patients to comply with radiation safety precautions, uncontrolled hyperthyroidism, and active thyroid orbitopathy.

3.1. Graves' disease

Graves' disease patients in iodine-sufficient areas are approximately 80% of patients with thyrotoxicosis or hyperthyroidism [8]. Graves' disease, also known as toxic diffuse goiter, is an autoimmune disease characterized by elevated levels of TSH receptor antibodies with increased production of thyroid hormones. TSH receptor antibodies bind to the TSH receptor and stimulate it chronically, which results in thyroid gland function becoming autonomous and independent of TSH feedback.

In general, Graves' disease therapeutic options are ATDs, RAI, and surgery. Thus, a therapeutic strategy should be individualized in patient considering several situations such as patient's clinical characteristics, age, and life style of the patient. ATDs are the most common treatment especially in children, teenagers, and pregnant women and also ATDs should be used as a first-line therapy to have the patient in euthyroidal status before the choice of treatment.

Commonly, methimazole is the first option drug, although propylthiouracil may be administrated in rare cases. ATDs' key adverse effects are rash, artralgy, agranulocytosis, and hepatitis. The usual ATDs administration should be for 6–18 months and time to initial improvements are 2–4 weeks. However, in about half of the patients relapse of hyperthyroidism may be experienced when the ATDs are withdrawn after a standard 1–2 years of therapy [9].

Surgery is usually preferred in cases of large goiters with compressive symptoms or during second trimester of pregnancy. However, hospitalization and surgery complications including hypoparathyroidism and recurrent laryngeal nerve injury and also anesthesia complications can be practiced.

RAI treatment is increasingly preferred in Graves' disease as first treatment and also after ATDs treatment or thyroid surgery in uncontrolled hyperthyroidism patients. Most patients are effectively treated with a single therapeutic dose of RAI. The symptoms of hyperthyroidism are expected to improve within 3 weeks of therapy; yet, the therapeutic effect takes 3–6 months because of the stored thyroid hormone to be released [10]. However, RAI therapy may not be effective in approximately 10% of patients [10]. In these patients, the repeat RAI treatment can be administered and usually the administered repeat dose should be of similar or higher than the first dose of RAI.

3.2. Toxic nodular goiter

Toxic nodular goiter (TNG) is the second most common cause of hyperthyroidism, after Graves' disease [11], which may be presented with toxic multinodular goiter (TMNG) also known as Plummer's disease or solitary hyperfunctioning nodule, also known as toxic adenoma. Hyperthyroidism may occur in both presentations. TNG autonomously produces excess thyroid hormones, resulting in hyperthyroidism. TSH receptor mutations in TNG have been reported to be as high as 80%. Somatic activating mutations of the TSH receptor activate the cAMP pathway and cause clonal autonomous growth and hyperfunctioning of the thyroid follicular cells, which results in TNG.

Toxic nodules are more resistant to RAI therapy than Graves' disease [10]. Considering this fact, the administered therapeutic RAI dose is often increased by 50% compared to what would be given in Graves' disease.

3.3. I131 induced hyperthyroidism

Excessive I131 exposure, usually following the use of I131 containing drugs such as amiodarone, expectorants, and contrast agents, is the main cause of I131-induced hyperthyroidism and can cause destructive thyroiditis. The symptoms are similar to autoimmune thyroiditis, but because of the long biologic half-life of amiodarone and its metabolites the symptoms, it lasts longer. High I131 may induce increased synthesis of thyroid hormone, known as Jod-Basedow, usually occurring in nodular thyroid glands and is more common in endemic goiter areas. It can be treated with ATDs and also combination of potassium perchlorate may help to decrease thyroidal iodine content. Persistent cases may be treated with RAI definitively if the thyroid uptake is adequate, provided that the agent has been discontinued for sufficient time of up to 2 years (mean period of 6 months) for the excess iodine load to be eliminated [12].

4. Patient preparation

Radioiodine therapy for patients with thyroid disease requires close cooperation between the nuclear medicine physician and the endocrinologist. The assurance of adequate therapy conditions is the overall responsibility of the nuclear medicine physician.

Evaluation of the patient before RAI therapy should include previous treatment of the patient (e.g., use of ATDs, amiodarone, contrast media, other iodine-containing medication, and iodine-containing food) and laboratory testing, including free T4, free T3, and TSH [13]. Thyroid scan preferably with I123, otherwise with Tc-99m, may be acquired.

Before RAI therapy, RAI uptake test should be performed for the differential diagnosis of hyperthyroidism to determine the I131 usage by the thyroid gland, and the calculation of the treatment dose. Increased RAI uptake values in patients with hyperthyroidism shows that elevated thyroid hormones belong to hyperfunctioning thyroid gland [14].

The 24-hour thyroid uptake in Graves' disease is generally high; on the other hand, it is often normal or mildly elevated in TNG. RAI uptake test level obtained at 24-hour should be greater than 20%. If this level is lower than 20%, other treatment methods should be considered [13].

Thyroid gland volume and intrathoracic thyroid extension assessment should be acquired by ultrasonography. In patients with large goiters, intrathoracic extension can be evaluated with thyroid scan with sternal notch marked, magnetic resonance imaging, or computed tomography. If the evaluation is held with radiocontrast computed tomography, it should be kept in mind that radiocontrast agents will reduce the radioiodine uptake for weeks to months and as such disabling radioiodine therapy during that time.

The nodules larger than 1–1.5 cm with a suspicious ultrasonographic look with nonfunctioning cold scan appearance in the thyroid scan should be assessed by fine needle aspiration biopsy to rule out malignancy.

The status of eye disease should be examined in patients with Graves' ophthalmopathy by an experienced ophthalmologist.

In patients with severe thyrotoxicosis with high risk of thyroid storm and elderly patients should be maintained in euthyroidism status with ATDs, preferably with methimazole.

And treatment of other comorbid diseases should be regulated.

Patients receiving more than 444 MBq of RAI for benign thyroid diseases have dose rates of 0.02 mSv per hour at 1 meter and so precautions are imposed. They do not require isolation, but they have to be cautioned to avoid contact with children and pregnant women, to sleep alone, to flush the toilet two to three times after use, and use separate utensils for 2–4 days and the effects of time and distance on dose should be indicated.

All patients receiving RAI should be given clear information about the treatment as well as written instructions for relevant precautions to avoid exposing others to unnecessary irradiation after treatment. Female patients in child bearing age and during pregnancy must be excluded and these patients should be counseled to avoid pregnancy for 3–6 months and to use contraception for 4 months after therapy.

5. I131 dose selection

Generally, the dose of RAI depends on the gland size, RAI uptake test, and biologic half-life of RAI in the thyroid gland [15], which may widely differ; however, several methods have been experienced for selecting adequate dose of RAI therapy in patients with hyperfunctioning thyroid gland [10].

A standard dose of 185–555 MBq is often prescribed. Yet, large glands need a relatively higher therapeutic dose and patients with a high RAI uptake test results need a lower dose.

Another method is using a standard formula with gland size, the RAI uptake test, and the proposed administered I131 dose per gram of thyroid tissue. Thus, an individual therapy dose for each patient is calculated by using the following formula [10]:

$$\text{I131 administered dose} = \frac{\text{Gram size of thyroid gland} \times 100-180\ \mu\text{Ci/g}}{\text{24 hour \% RAI uptake}} \quad (1)$$

Another approach is to calculate the MBq per gram dose. The patients with nodular goiters and patients with very large toxic diffuse goiters are often referred for repeated therapies. In this method, the referring physician often prefers the higher dose (4.44–6.66 MBq/g tissue) for a higher likelihood of success with a single therapeutic dose.

Moreover, a higher RAI dose requirement is needed in patients, with a 4-hour I131 uptake result exceeding the 24-hour I131 uptake result, suggesting the rapid iodine turnover [15, 16].

6. Special conditions

6.1. Withdrawal of antithyroid drugs

ATDs are the initial treatment option for patients with hyperthyroidism. ATDs pretreatment diminishes thyroid hormone stores and therefore decreases the risk of thyrotoxicrisis and the aggravation of symptoms after RAI treatment, constituting a safe patient preparation for RAI treatment [17]. However, ATDs pretreatment may lead to undesirable effects, such as an increased risk of radioiodine failure and worsening of thyrotoxicosis after discontinuation for pretreatment of RAI [17, 18].

Even though some studies support that pretreatment of ATDs may reduce the effect of RAI treatment [19, 20], some studies claim that they have no obvious effect [21, 22]. This side effect of ATDs is the possible radioprotective effect that seems to depend on a sulphhydryl group contained in ATDs. On the other hand, ATDs such as methimazole and carbimazole, which do not possess sulphhydryl groups and may be, do not possess radioprotective effect either [23]. Thus, pretreatment with thiouracils has been shown to reduce the therapeutic effectiveness of RAI, but the usage of carbimazole or methimazole has not been observed with similar effect [24]. This negative impact on RAI treatment can be compensated by discontinuation of the medication before RAI administration if the patient can tolerate it. Pretreatment with propyl-thiouracil (PTU) is stopped for at least 2–3 weeks (if possible 8 weeks) before RAI treatment is given due to radioprotective effect of PTU [13]. Owing to methimazole and carbimazole having no side effect on cure rate, these drugs are stopped a few days before planned RAI administration [25, 26]. Beta-adrenergic antagonists (usually propranolol) can be used as an alternative to control hyperthyroidism symptoms during ATDs withdrawal. After RAI administration, ATDs should be restarted from the same recommended dose before RAI treatment. ATDs do not have to be restarted in young patients or in patients with mild hyperthyroidism.

6.2. Lithium usage

Lithium can block RAI release from the thyroid but does not interfere with RAI uptake. In general, lithium pretreatment is not routinely recommended but its administration can be considered for 7 days if 24-hour RAI uptake test is less than 20% [27]. However, a randomized controlled trial has found no evidence of an effect of lithium on RAI therapy when it is given for a few days after RAI treatment. The authors commented as it may increase the efficiency of RAI, but this effect is unclear [28]. Another research showed that lithium treatment prevents the rise in serum thyroid hormones after withdrawal of ATDs for RAI therapy [29].

6.3. Recombinant human TSH (rhTSH)

Recombinant human TSH (rhTSH; Thyrogen, Genzyme Transgenics Corp.) is developed to provide TSH stimulation without withdrawal of thyroid hormones. The therapeutic effect of I131 in patients with nodular goiter depends to some extent on the RAI uptake. The main cause of a low RAI uptake in patients with TNG is normal or below normal serum TSH levels. In patients with nontoxic or TNG with low I131 uptake, the administration of rhTSH increases

RAI uptake significantly and retention in the thyroid gland and minimizes the radiation dose to the remainder of the body without increase in serum thyroid hormones levels [15, 30]. Besides, by stimulating I131 uptake in relatively cold areas, more than in relatively hot areas, a more homogeneous distribution of I131 within the thyroid gland is observed in patients with nodular goiter, after single low dose rhTSH administration [31].

For the optimization of rhTSH dose, different rhTSH doses have been utilized. A study showed that a dose of 0.01 mg rhTSH administered 24 hours before RAI increases 24-hour RAIU from 29 to 51%, while 0.03 mg rhTSH increased 24-hour RAIU from 33 to 63% [32]. Another study presented that RAI treatment after the administration of a single, low dose of rhTSH in patients with nodular goiter resulted in thyroid volume reduction 1 year after treatment by 35% in the group pretreated with 0.01 mg rhTSH and by 41% in the group pretreated with 0.03 mg rhTSH [33].

The leading side effects in nodular goiter are sensation of thyroidal swelling, transient thyroiditis, and transient goiter volume enlargement, which may lead to a significant cervical compression within the first month of treatment after the administration of 0.3 mg of rhTSH [34].

In the adjunct therapies with very small doses of rhTSH (0.03–0.1 mg) in patients with multinodular goiter, either they were euthyroid or hyperthyroid, few safety concerns have been observed [35, 36]. Currently, the adjunct therapy with rhTSH is not indicated in patients with TMNG because of the risk of exacerbating patient's hyperthyroidism [37].

7. Precautions for RAI therapy

The RAI preparations have negligible content of 0.05–0.18 μg large stable I131, which is much lower than the average daily iodine intake [13]. Therefore, even patients with known I131 sensitivity can be treated with RAI safely.

On the other hand, approximately 7 days following RAI administration, temporary increase in serum thyroid hormone levels may be expected. Hence, RAI is contraindicated in patients who has uncontrolled symptoms of hyperthyroidism or high levels of free T3. The elevation of thyroid hormones may trigger atrial fibrillation or heart failure, leading to thyroid storm. These patients should continue using ATDs and beta-blockers for symptomatic control. Likewise, beta-blockers need not be stopped before RAI treatment. But, if ATDs are contraindicated (e.g., due to agranulocytosis or posttherapy liver failure) and surgery cannot be performed due to symptoms of hyperthyroidism, RAI may be given under steroid treatment (usually hydrocortisone 50–100 mg i.v.) and beta-blockers [13].

Similarly, patients with large nodular goiters should be treated under steroid treatment to prevent RAI-induced swelling thyroid, which rarely aggravates airway obstruction.

7.1. Graves' ophthalmopathy

Graves' disease exophthalmos cannot be controlled by ATDs and RAI therapy [38]. Furthermore, RAI may cause progression of Graves' ophthalmopathy. After RAI therapy, 15% of the patients with Graves' disease may acquire newly evolving Graves' ophthalmopathy [39] and up to 39% of patients may experience worsening of the former ophthalmopathy within 6 months [40].

The risk factors for progression of Graves' ophthalmopathy are preexisting ophthalmopathy, smoking [41], high levels of pretreatment serumT3 and TSH receptor antibody and thyrotropin receptor antibody levels (>7.5 IU/L) [42], severity of hyperthyroidism, and post-RAI hypothyroidism [38, 43, 44].

Thus, all patients who will receive RAI treatment should first be maintained in euthyroid state with ATDs and should be advised to quit smoking because of the increased risk of evolving of ophthalmopathy in smokers after RAI therapy [45]. The use of ATDs does not seem to be associated with the developing or worsening of preexisting ophthalmopathy in patients with Graves' disease [46]. In patients with active ophthalmopathy, the risk can be reduced by a short cycle (3 months) of oral prednisone (0.3–0.5 mg/kg/d) started 1–3 days following RAI therapy and continued for 1 month, with tapering over the subsequent 2 months and by avoiding post-RAI hypothyroidism with synthetic thyroid hormone placement [38, 43]. Despite the widespread usage of steroid prophylaxis, its optimal schedule is undefined. The European Group on Graves' Orbitopathy (EUGOGO) Consensus Statement on management of Graves' ophthalmopathy suggested that a shorter term (about 2 months) of oral steroids treatment might be equally protective [38]. A recent retrospective cohort study suggested that starting from a few days after RAI therapy, 0.2 mg/kg/day of oral prednisolone for 6 weeks may be effective in preventing RAI-associated progression of Graves' ophthalmopathy [47].

Patients with inactive Graves' ophthalmopathy, if they do not have the risk factors for Graves' ophthalmopathy, can have RAI therapy without steroid coverage as long as hypothyroidism is avoided [38].

8. Adverse effect of I131 therapy

The common acute side effects in the gastrointestinal tract are heartburn, nausea, diarrhea, and vomiting.

The acute adverse effects of RAI therapy include radiation-induced thyroiditis that is associated with neck pain thyroid swelling and transient thyrotoxicosis. Thyroid swelling may appear after a few days following the therapy. The symptoms can be managed by nonsteroidal antiinflammatory drug. Early after RAI therapy, even though the goiter volume and the impact on the respiratory function remain unchanged [48], the critical thyroid swelling and respiratory distress can be experienced, fortunately it is a rare complication [49]. If the presence of tracheal compression is previously known, especially in large goiter patients, 25 mg prednisolone may be given daily for 14 days to prevent thyroid swelling from RAI therapy [48].

Transient thyrotoxicosis, a transient elevation of the thyroid hormone levels, can be practiced due to the secretion of stored hormones from the thyroid gland. Thyroid storm or thyrotoxicrisis is a rare but severe and potentially life-threatening hypermetabolic condition induced by excessive release of thyroid hormones. The treatment must include i.v. infusion of ATDs, steroids, and beta-blockers to avoid a fatal outcome.

Other side effects of RAI therapy include sialoadenitis leading to temporary or permanent salivary gland dysfunction and lacrimal canal obstruction, which can be demonstrated as RAI-induced acute histopathological changes as well. Hydration should be encouraged to minimize these problems. Sour candy can be suggested for salivary gland dysfunction. However, there are also studies demonstrating that permanent xerostomia is significantly more common in patients having sour candy in the first 24 hours of RAI therapy than in patients having the candy after the first day [50]. Consequently, several antioxidant agents are under evaluation to reduce these changes in many researches [51–53].

The main and long-term adverse effect of RAI therapy is the hypothyroidism. Usually in the first 2 years after RAI therapy, hypothyroidism occurs in up to 50% of patients and the risk increases in patients with small goiter size, positive TPO antibodies, and a family history of autoimmune thyroid disease [54]. Pretreatment of ATDs does not affect the frequency of hypothyroidism. Generally, it is very difficult to predict if the development of hypothyroidism is either transient or permanent. In a few months after RAI therapy, if the level of serum TSH is still above 45 mU/L, transient hypothyroidism is ruled out [55]. A transient hypothyroidism develops a few months after RAI therapy and continues about 1–4 months and does not require thyroid hormones replacement. The patients should be offered annual follow-up testing of thyroid hormones.

Another adverse effect is the post-RAI autoimmune thyroiditis and immunogenic hyperthyroidism/Graves' disease. About 1% of patients following RAI therapy of nodular goiter may develop Graves' disease. This risk increases approximately 10-fold when TPO antibody levels are elevated before RAI. The release of thyroid antigens and other immunogenic effects of RAI on thyroid-autoreactive lymphocytes are the presumed mechanisms. In addition, there is an estimated 1.3% risk of a temporary increase of TSH receptor antibodies after RAI for autonomous thyroid disease without the development of clinically apparent hyperthyroidism [56].

Finally, even though, the chromosomal damage in peripheral lymphocytes is induced after RAI therapy for benign thyroid diseases [57], the role of I131 in radiation-induced cancers remains unclear. There is no evidence of the risk of malignancy as a consequence of thyroid and whole-body irradiation. Though there is low risk of preexisting or coexisting thyroid cancer in patients with toxic nodular goiter and Graves' disease unrelated to RAI therapy [58].

9. Results

The success of RAI therapy is defined as the elimination of hyperthyroidism, in which the patient may be either in euthyroid state or in hypothyroid state that is compensated by synthetic thyroid hormone. The successful therapy rate depends on thyroid volume, compensation of hyperthyroidism, I131 intake in the diet, the timing of the withdrawal of ATDs, and the dosage in the different thyroid diseases.

The low fixed activity (185 MBq) of I131 seems to be effective in 73% of Indian patients with Graves' disease, 1 year after RAI therapy [59]. Another study compared doses of 370 and 555 MBq of RAI and the success rates at 12 months of both doses brought about a similar remission of the hyperthyroidism in patients with Graves' disease [27, 60].

A study based on tissue-absorbed dose calculations demonstrated that the frequency of persistent hyperthyroidism decreased to 27% after 150 Gy, to 23% after 200 Gy, and to 8% after 300 Gy [61]. However, the possibility of occurrence of hypothyroidism increases over years and patients need to be in regular follow-up.

RAI therapy is more successful in patients with nodules smaller than 2 cm [62]. However, there is currently no consensus about the appropriate RAI dose in TNG, both the fixed dose or calculated dose can be given. Effect of fixed and calculated doses on hyperthyroidism was compared in a meta-analysis that reported both methods to be equally successful [63].

Zakavi et al. compared fixed low and fixed high RAI doses for treating a single toxic thyroid nodule in patients with no age, sex ratio, thyroid uptake, and thyroid weight differences. Ten months after RAI therapy, the success of hyperthyroidism treatment was higher in patients calculated with high dose therapy than other groups [64].

Glucocorticoids did not influence the final outcome following RAI [65]. At least 2 days of methimazole withdrawal was long enough to restore the success of RAI therapy [26].

10. Follow-up

After the RAI administration ATDs should be restarted after 3–5 days and withdrawn as soon as thyroid function normalizes and synthetic thyroid hormone replacement should be started as soon as hypothyroidism occurs [8].

Patients who have been given RAI therapy should be essentially followed up in regular review of thyroid function tests to evaluate the effectiveness of the treatment and for timely detection of developing hypothyroidism or posttreatment immunogenic hyperthyroidism. Follow-up should be basically performed with TSH and serum T4 tests, 4–6 weeks after RAI treatment. The patients receiving ATDs or having increased risk of developing or worsening of Graves' ophthalmopathy due to hypothyroidism, shorter intervals of the tests should be performed 2–3 weeks after RAI treatment is recommended [13]. All the patients should have annual laboratory tests, at least TSH levels should be checked regularly. In patients with relapse or persistent hyperthyroidism, RAI treatment can be repeated after 6–12 months.

11. Conclusion

With over 7 decades of experience, RAI therapy is an individualized, safe, and effective treatment modality, which is doubtlessly going to be still available in the future with possible up coming features in genetics.

In several types of hyperthyroidism TSH receptor gene mutations may be expressed, for instance, familial gestational hyperthyroidism, autonomous toxic adenomas, hereditary or sporadic toxic thyroid hyperplasia, familial nonautoimmune hyperthyroidism, and Graves' disease. Genetic studies focusing on the mutations of TSH receptor gene and their alterations with the related genes would probably open a new door in the understanding of the process and may support the prospective treatments.

In addition to safeguard the other tissues especially nonthyroidal NIS-expressing tissues, e.g., lactating breast, gastric mucosa, lacrimal glands, and salivary glands, for example, temporarily opening tissue-specific NIS expression or downregulating the functional expression of NIS in different cellular models may certainly provide an optimal use by directly affecting the RAI dose received by the specific target tissue [66].

Author details

Aylin Akbulut*, Fadimana Nur Aydinbelge and Gökhan Koca

*Address all correspondence to: aylinbaskin@gmail.com

Department of Nuclear Medicine, Ankara Training and Research Hospital, University of Health Sciences, Ankara, Turkey

References

[1] Hertz S, Roberts A. Radioactive iodine in the study of thyroid physiology; the use of radioactive iodine therapy in hyperthyroidism. Journal of the American Medical Association. 1946;**131**:81-86. DOİ: 10.1001/jama.1946.02870190005002

[2] Bender JM, Dworkin HJ. Therapy of hyperthyroidism. In: Henkin RE, editor. Nuclear Medicine. 1st ed. Missouri: Mosby; 1996. pp. 1549-1567

[3] Spitzweg C, Morris JC. The sodium iodide symporter: Its pathophysiological and therapeutic implications. Clinical Endocrinology. 2002;**57**(5):559-574. DOI: 10.1046/j.1365-2265.2002.01640.x

[4] Castro MR, Bergert ER, Beito TG, McIver B, Goellner JR, Morris JC. Development of monoclonal antibodies against the human sodium iodide symporter: Immunohistochemical characterization of this protein in thyroid cells 1. The Journal of Clinical Endocrinology & Metabolism. 1999;**84**(8):2957-2962. DOİ: 10.1677/joe.0.1630495

[5] Joba W, Spitzweg C, Schriever K, Heufelder AE. Analysis of human sodium/iodide symporter, thyroid transcription factor-1, and paired-box-protein-8 gene expression in benign thyroid diseases. Thyroid. 1999;**9**(5):455-466. DOI: 10.1089/thy.1999.9.455

[6] Caillou B, Troalen F, Baudin E, Talbot M, Filetti S, Schlumberger M, et al. Na^+/I^- Symporter distribution in human thyroid tissues: An Immunohistochemical study 1. The Journal of Clinical Endocrinology & Metabolism. 1998;**83**(11):4102-4106. DOI: 10.1210/jcem.83.11.5262

[7] Dobyns BM, Vickery AL, Maloof F, Chapman EM. Functional and histologic effects of therapeutic doses of radioactive iodine on the thyroid of man. The Journal of Clinical Endocrinology and Metabolism. 1953;**13**(5):548-567

[8] De Leo S, Lee SY, Braverman LE. Hyperthyroidism. Lancet. 2016;**388**(10047):906-918. DOI: 10.1016/S0140-6736(16)00278-6

[9] Laurberg P, Krejbjerg A, Andersen SL. Relapse following antithyroid drug therapy for Graves' hyperthyroidism. Current Opinion in Endocrinology, Diabetes, and Obesity. 2014;**21**(5):415-421. DOİ: 10.1097/MED.0000000000000088

[10] Ziessman HA, O'Malley JP, Thrall JH, editors. Nuclear Medicine: The Requisites. 3rd ed. Philadelphia: Elsevier Mosby; 2006. pp. 71-101. ISBN: 978-0323-02946946-9

[11] Nayak B, Hodak SP. Hyperthyroidism. Endocrinology & Metabolism Clinics of North America. 2007;**36**(3):617-656. v. DOI: 10.1016/j.ecl.2007.06.002

[12] Eskes SA, Wiersinga WM. Amiodarone and thyroid. Best Practice & Research Clinical Endocrinology & Metabolism. 2009;**23**(6):735-751. DOİ: 10.1016/j.beem.2009.07.001

[13] Stokkel MP, Junak DH, Lassmann M, Dietlein M, Luster M. EANM procedure guidelines for therapy of benign thyroid disease. European Journal of Nuclear Medicine and Molecular Imaging. 2010;**37**(11):2218-2228. DOI: 10.1007/s00259-010-1536-8

[14] Sarkar SD. Benign thyroid disease: What is the role of nuclear medicine? Seminars in Nuclear Medicine. 2006;**36**(3):185-193. DOI: 10.1053/j.semnuclmed.2006.03.006

[15] Silberstein EB, Alavi A, Balon HR, Clarke SE, Divgi C, Gelfand MJ, et al. The SNMMI practice guideline for therapy of thyroid disease with 131I 3.0. Journal of Nuclear Medicine. 2012;**53**(10):1633-1651. DOİ: 10.2967/jnumed.112.105148

[16] Isgoren S, Daglioz Gorur G, Demir H, Berk F. Radioiodine therapy in Graves' disease: Is it possible to predict outcome before therapy? Nuclear Medicine Communications. 2012;**33**(8):859-863. DOI: 10.1097/MNM.0b013e3283559ba1

[17] Burch H, Solomon B, Cooper D, Ferguson P, Walpert N, Howard R. The effect of antithyroid drug pretreatment on acute changes in thyroid hormone levels after 131I ablation for Graves' disease 1. The Journal of Clinical Endocrinology & Metabolism. 2001;**86**(7):3016-3021. DOI: https://doi.org/10.1210/jcem.86.7.7639

[18] Hancock LD, Tuttle RM, LeMar H, Bauman J, Patience T. The effect of propylthiouracil on subsequent radioactive iodine therapy in Graves' disease. Clinical Endocrinology. 1997;**47**(4):425-430. DOI: 10.1046/j.1365-2265.1997.2741075.x

[19] Crooks J, Buchanan WW, Wayne E, MacDonald E. Effect of pretreatment with methylthiouracil on results of 131I therapy. British Medical Journal. 1960;**1**(5167):151. DOI: 10.1136/bmj.1.5167.151

[20] Reynolds LR, Kotchen TA. Antithyroid drugs and radioactive iodine: Fifteen years' experience with Graves' disease. Archives of Internal Medicine. 1979;**139**(6):651-653. DOI: 10.1530/eje.1.01904

[21] Goolden A, Fraser TR. Effect of pretreatment with carbimazole in patients with thyrotoxicosis subsequently treated with radioactive iodine. British Medical Journal. 1969;**3**(5668):443-444. DOI: 10.1136/bmj.3.5668.443

[22] Marcocci C, Gianchecchi D, Masini I, Golia F, Ceccarelli C, Bracci E, et al. A reappraisal of the role of methimazole and other factors on the efficacy and outcome of radioiodine therapy of Graves' hyperthyroidism. Journal of Endocrinological Investigation. 1990;**13**(6):513-520. DOI: 10.1007/BF03348615

[23] Moka D, Dietlein M, Schicha H. Radioiodine therapy and thyrostatic drugs and iodine. European Journal of Nuclear Medicine and Molecular Imaging. 2002;**29**(Suppl. 2):486-491. DOI: 10.1007/s00259-002-0868-4

[24] Imseis RE, Vanmiddlesworth L, Massie JD, Bush AJ, Vanmiddlesworth N. Pretreatment with propylthiouracil but not methimazole reduces the therapeutic efficacy of iodine-131 in hyperthyroidism. The Journal of Clinical Endocrinology & Metabolism. 1998;**83**(2):685-687. DOI: 10.1210/jcem.83.2.4538

[25] Andrade VA, Gross JL, Maia AL. The effect of methimazole pretreatment on the efficacy of radioactive iodine therapy in Graves' hyperthyroidism: One-year follow-up of a prospective, randomized study. The Journal of Clinical Endocrinology & Metabolism. 2001;**86**(8):3488-3493. DOI: 10.1210/jcem.86.8.7707

[26] Dunkelmann S, Kuenstner H, Nabavi E, Rohde B, Groth P, Schuemichen C. Change in the intrathyroidal kinetics of radioiodine under continued and discontinued antithyroid medication in Graves' disease. European Journal of Nuclear Medicine and Molecular Imaging. 2007;**34**(2):228-236. DOI: 10.1007/s00259-006-0234-z

[27] Bogazzi F, Bartalena L, Brogioni S, Scarcello G, Burelli A, Campomori A, et al. Comparison of radioiodine with radioiodine plus lithium in the treatment of Graves' hyperthyroidism 1. The Journal of Clinical Endocrinology & Metabolism. 1999;**84**(2):499-503. DOI: 10.1210/jcem.84.2.5446

[28] Bal C, Kumar A, Pandey R. A randomized controlled trial to evaluate the adjuvant effect of lithium on radioiodine treatment of hyperthyroidism. Thyroid: Official journal of the American Thyroid Association. 2002;**12**(5):399-405. DOI: 10.1089/105072502760043486

[29] Bogazzi F, Bartalena L, Campomori A, Brogioni S, Traino C, De Martino F, et al. Treatment with lithium prevents serum thyroid hormone increase after thionamide withdrawal and radioiodine therapy in patients with Graves' disease. The Journal of Clinical Endocrinology & Metabolism. 2002;**87**(10):4490-4495. DOI: 10.1210/jc.2002-020580.

[30] Braverman L, Kloos R, Law Jr B, Kipnes M, Dionne M, Magner J. Evaluation of various doses of recombinant human thyrotropin in patients with multinodular goiters. Endocrine Practice. 2008;**14**(7):832-839. DOI: 10.4158/EP.14.7.832

[31] Nieuwlaat WA, Hermus AR, Sivro-Prndelj F, Corstens FH, Huysmans DA. Pretreatment with recombinant human TSH changes the regional distribution of radioiodine on thyroid scintigrams of nodular goiters. The Journal of Clinical Endocrinology and Metabolism. 2001;**86**(11):5330-5336. DOI: 10.1210/jcem.86.11.8014

[32] Huysmans DA, Nieuwlaat WA, Erdtsieck RJ, Schellekens AP, Bus JW, Bravenboer B, et al. Administration of a single low dose of recombinant human thyrotropin significantly enhances thyroid radioiodide uptake in nontoxic nodular goiter. The Journal of Clinical Endocrinology and Metabolism. 2000;**85**(10):3592-3596. DOI: 10.1210/jcem.85.10.6869

[33] Nieuwlaat WA, Huysmans DA, van den Bosch HC, Sweep CG, Ross HA, Corstens FH, et al. Pretreatment with a single, low dose of recombinant human thyrotropin allows dose reduction of radioiodine therapy in patients with nodular goiter. The Journal of Clinical Endocrinology and Metabolism. 2003;**88**(7):3121-3129. DOI: 10.1210/jc.2002-021554

[34] Nielsen VE, Bonnema SJ, Hegedus L. Transient goiter enlargement after administration of 0.3 mg of recombinant human thyrotropin in patients with benign nontoxic nodular goiter: A randomized, double-blind, crossover trial. The Journal of Clinical Endocrinology and Metabolism. 2006;**91**(4):1317-1322. DOI: 10.1210/jc.2005-2137

[35] Graf H, Fast S, Pacini F, Pinchera A, Leung A, Vaisman M, et al. Modified-release recombinant human TSH (MRrhTSH) augments the effect of (131)I therapy in benign multinodular goiter: Results from a multicenter international, randomized, placebo-controlled study. The Journal of Clinical Endocrinology and Metabolism. 2011;**96**(5):1368-1376. DOI: 10.1210/jc.2010-1193

[36] Paz-Filho GJ, Mesa-Junior CO, Olandoski M, Woellner LC, Goedert CA, Boguszewski CL, et al. Effect of 30 mCi radioiodine on multinodular goiter previously treated with recombinant human thyroid-stimulating hormone. Brazilian Journal of Medical and Biological Research = Revista brasileira de pesquisas medicas e biologicas. 2007;**40**(12):1661-1670. DOI: 10.1590/S0100-879X2006005000186

[37] Bahn Chair RS, Burch HB, Cooper DS, Garber JR, Greenlee MC, Klein I, et al. Hyperthyroidism and other causes of thyrotoxicosis: Management guidelines of the American Thyroid Association and American Association of Clinical Endocrinologists. Thyroid: Official Journal of the American Thyroid Association. 2011;**21**(6):593-646. DOI: 10.1089/thy.2010.0417

[38] Bartalena L, Baldeschi L, Dickinson A, Eckstein A, Kendall-Taylor P, Marcocci C, et al. Consensus statement of the European Group on Graves' orbitopathy (EUGOGO) on management of GO. European Journal of Endocrinology. 2008;**158**(3):273-285. DOI: 10.1530/EJE-07-0666

[39] Vannucchi G, Campi I, Covelli D, Dazzi D, Currò N, Simonetta S, et al. Graves' Orbitopathy activation after radioactive iodine therapy with and without steroid prophylaxis. The Journal of Clinical Endocrinology & Metabolism. 2009;**94**(9):3381-3386. DOI: 10.1210/jc.2009-0506

[40] Traisk F, Tallstedt L, Abraham-Nordling M, Andersson T, Berg G, Calissendorff J, et al. Thyroid-associated ophthalmopathy after treatment for Graves' hyperthyroidism with antithyroid drugs or iodine-131. The Journal of Clinical Endocrinology and Metabolism. 2009;**94**(10):3700-3707. DOI: 10.1210/jc.2009-0747

[41] Bartalena L, Marcocci C, Tanda ML, Manetti L, Dell'Unto E, Bartolomei MP, et al. Cigarette smoking and treatment outcomes in Graves ophthalmopathy. Annals of internal medicine. 1998;**129**(8):632-635. DOI: 10.7326/0003-4819-129-8-199810150-00010

[42] Eckstein AK, Plicht M, Lax H, Neuhäuser M, Mann K, Lederbogen S, et al. Thyrotropin receptor autoantibodies are independent risk factors for Graves' ophthalmopathy and help to predict severity and outcome of the disease. The Journal of Clinical Endocrinology & Metabolism. 2006;**91**(9):3464-3470. DOI: 10.1210/jc.2005-2813

[43] Bartalena L, Marcocci C, Bogazzi F, Manetti L, Tanda ML, Dell'Unto E, et al. Relation between therapy for hyperthyroidism and the course of Graves' ophthalmopathy. New England Journal of Medicine. 1998;**338**(2):73-78. DOI: 10.1056/NEJM199801083380201

[44] Ponto KA, Zang S, Kahaly GJ. The tale of radioiodine and Graves' orbitopathy. Thyroid: Official journal of the American Thyroid Association. 2010;**20**(7):785-793. DOI: 10.1089/thy.2010.1640

[45] Acharya SH, Avenell A, Philip S, Burr J, Bevan JS, Abraham P. Radioiodine therapy (RAI) for Graves' disease (GD) and the effect on ophthalmopathy: A systematic review. Clinical Endocrinology. 2008;69(6):943-950. DOI: 10.1111/j.1365-2265.2008.03279.x

[46] Prummel MF, Wiersinga WM, Mounts MP, Koornneef L, Berghout A, van der Gaag R. Effect of abnormal thyroid function on the severity of Graves' ophthalmopathy. Archives of Internal Medicine. 1990;**150**(5):1098-1101. DOI: 10.1001/archinte.1990.00390170124027

[47] Lai A, Sassi L, Compri E, Marino F, Sivelli P, Piantanida E, et al. Lower dose prednisone prevents radioiodine-associated exacerbation of initially mild or absent Graves' orbitopathy: A retrospective cohort study. The Journal of Clinical Endocrinology & Metabolism. 2010;**95**(3):1333-1337. DOI: 10.1210/jc.2009-2130

[48] Bonnema SJ, Fast S, Hegedüs L. The role of radioiodine therapy in benign nodular goitre. Best Practice & Research Clinical Endocrinology & Metabolism. 2014;**28**(4):619-631. DOI: 10.1016/j.beem.2014.02.001

[49] Kinuya S, Yoneyama T, Michigishi T. Airway complication occurring during radioiodine treatment for Graves' disease. Annals of Nuclear Medicine. 2007;**21**(6):367-369. DOI: 10.1007/s12149-007-0034-y

[50] Nakada K, Ishibashi T, Takei T, Hirata K, Shinohara K, Katoh S, et al. Does lemon candy decrease salivary gland damage after radioiodine therapy for thyroid cancer? Journal of Nuclear Medicine. 2005;**46**(2):261-266

[51] Koca G, Gültekin SS, Han Ü, Kuru S, Demirel K, Korkmaz M. The efficacy of montelukast as a protective agent against 131I-induced salivary gland damage in rats: Scintigraphic and histopathological findings. Nuclear Medicine Communications. 2013;**34**(5):507-517. DOI: 10.1097/MNM.0b013e32835ffecd

[52] Acar DE, Acar U, Yumusak N, Korkmaz M, Acar M, Atilgan HI, et al. Reducing the histopathological changes of radioiodine to the lacrimal glands by a popular anti-oxidant: Lycopene. Current Eye Research. 2014;**39**(7):659-665. DOI: 10.3109/02713683.2013.867354

[53] Acar U, Atilgan HI, Acar DE, Yalniz-Akkaya Z, Yumusak N, Korkmaz M, et al. The effect of short-term vitamin E against radioiodine-induced early lacrimal gland damage. Annals of Nuclear Medicine. 2013;**27**(10):886-891. DOI: 10.1007/s12149-013-0763-z

[54] Le Moli R, Wesche M, Tiel-van Buul M, Wiersinga W. Determinants of longterm outcome of radioiodine therapy of sporadic non-toxic goitre. Clinical Endocrinology (Oxford).. 1999;**50**:783-790. DOI: 10.1046/j.1365-2265.1999.00734.x

[55] Gómez N, Gómez JM, Orti A, Gavaldà L, Villabona C, Leyes P, et al. Transient hypothyroidism after iodine-131 therapy for Grave's disease. Journal Nuclear Medicine. 1995;**36**(9):1539-1542

[56] Schmidt M, Gorbauch E, Dietlein M, Faust M, Stützer H, Eschner W, et al. Incidence of postradioiodine immunogenic hyperthyroidism/Graves' disease in relation to a temporary increase in thyrotropin receptor antibodies after radioiodine therapy for autonomous thyroid disease. Thyroid. 2006;**16**(3):281-288. DOI: 10.1089/thy.2006.16.281

[57] Gutiérrez S, Carbonell E, Galofré P, Creus A, Marcos R. Cytogenetic damage after 131-iodine treatment for hyperthyroidism and thyroid cancer. European Journal of Nuclear Medicine and Molecular Imaging. 1999;**26**(12):1589-1596. DOI: 10.1007/s002590050499

[58] Ron E, Doody MM, Becker DV, Brill AB, Curtis RE, Goldman MB, et al. Cancer mortality following treatment for adult hyperthyroidism. Journal of the American Medical Association. 1998;**280**(4):347-355. DOI: 10.1001/jama.280.4.347

[59] Sanyal D, Mukhhopadhyay P, Pandit K, Chatterjee J, Raychaudhuri M, Mukherjee S, et al. Early treatment with low fixed dose (5 mCi) radioiodine therapy is effective in Indian subjects with Graves' disease. Journal of the Indian Medical Association. 2008;**106**(6):360-361, 72

[60] Canadas V, Vilar L, Moura E, Brito A, Castellar Ê. Evaluation of radioiodine therapy with fixed doses of 10 and 15 mCi in patients with graves disease. Arquivos Brasileiros de Endocrinologia & Metabologia. 2007;**51**(7):1069-1076. DOI: 10.1590/S0004-27302007000700008

[61] Reinhardt MJ, Brink I, Joe AY, von Mallek D, Ezziddin S, Palmedo H, et al. Radioiodine therapy in Graves' disease based on tissue-absorbed dose calculations: Effect of pretreatment thyroid volume on clinical outcome. European Journal of Nuclear Medicine and Molecular Imaging. 2002;**29**(9):1118-1124. DOI: 10.1007/s00259-002-0877-3

[62] Saki H, Cengiz A, Yurekli Y. Effectiveness of radioiodine treatment for toxic nodular goiter. Molecular Imaging and Radionuclide Therapy. 2015;**24**(3):100-104. DOI: 10.4274/mirt.48378

[63] de Rooij A, Vandenbroucke J, Smit J, Stokkel M, Dekkers O. Clinical outcomes after estimated versus calculated activity of radioiodine for the treatment of hyperthyroidism: Systematic review and meta-analysis. European Journal of Endocrinology. 2009;**161**(5):771-777. DOI: 10.1530/EJE-09-0286

[64] Zakavi SR, Mousavi Z, Davachi B. Comparison of four different protocols of I-131 therapy for treating single toxic thyroid nodule. Nuclear Medicine Communications. 2009;**30**(2):169-175. DOI: 10.1097/MNM.0b013e3283169148

[65] Jensen BE, Bonnema SJ, Hegedüs L. Glucocorticoids do not influence the effect of radioiodine therapy in Graves' disease. European Journal of Endocrinology. 2005;**153**(1):15-21. DOI: 10.1530/eje.1.01924

[66] Alotaibi H, Tuzlakoğlu-Öztürk M, Tazebay UH. The thyroid Na+/I-Symporter: Molecular characterization and genomic regulation. Molecular Imaging and Radionuclide Therapy. 2017; 26(Suppl 1): 92–101. DOI:10.4274/2017.26.suppl.11

Chapter 2

Radioiodine Therapy of Malignant Thyroid Diseases

Derya Cayir and Mine Araz

Additional information is available at the end of the chapter

http://dx.doi.org/10.5772/intechopen.68574

Abstract

Radioiodine-131 (I-131) is used in the treatment of thyroid diseases: hyperthyroidism and differentiated thyroid cancer (DTC: papillary, follicular, Hurthle cell cancer). Treatment success depends on several factors. The most fundamental factor affecting the success of treatment is the susceptibility to target tissue I-131. In patients with differentiated thyroid cancers following total thyroidectomy, I-131 is given for ablation of residual thyroid tissue and treatment of metastatic disease. Physical and biological characteristics of I-131, uptake and effect mechanisms of the iodine in the thyroid follicular cells, indications and contraindications for I-131 therapy, patient preparation and administration of I-131, follow-up and precautions on possible side effects, and an overview on the clinical studies about I-131 therapy are presented.

Keywords: iodine, thyroid diseases, therapeutics, radiation, neoplasms

1. Introduction

Radioiodine-131 (I-131) is successfully used in treatment of thyroid diseases: hyperthyroidism and differentiated thyroid cancer for several years. I-131 is available as sodium iodine in gelatine capsules and drinking solution for oral application and intravenous injections. Advantages of this therapy are good tolerability, easy application, safety, and efficacy of treatment. The critical organ for I-131 is the thyroid gland. I-131 is taken up by follicular cells. Retention of I-131 in the cells depends on the metabolic activity of the cells. I-131 simultaneously emits two types of radiation: beta minus (β^-) radiation used for the therapy and gamma (γ) used for diagnosis. Due to the penetration of beta particles in the tissue, damaging effect of β^- radiation is limited to thyroid cells. The physical and biological characteristics of I-131, uptake and effect mechanisms of the iodine in the thyroid follicular cells, indications and contraindications for I-131 therapy, patient preparation and administration of I-131, follow-up and precautions on possible side effects, and an overview on the clinical studies about I-131 therapy are presented under this title.

2. Epidemiology

Thyroid cancer constitutes 1.4% of all cancers and 15% of all endocrinologic malignancies. Thyroid cancer is responsible from 0.2 to 0.5% of cancer-related death. About 90–95% of thyroid cancers are differentiated thyroid cancers of follicular cell origin. Annual incidence is 1.2–2.6/100,000 in men and 2.0–3.8/100,000 in women. Mortality rates have been reported as 0.2–1.2/100,000 in men and 0.4–2.8/100,000 in women [1].

3. Treatment options: role of radioiodine

Front-line therapy of differentiated thyroid cancer (DTC) is surgery. Because multifocality and multicentricity is frequent, total or near-total thyroidectomy is the treatment of choice. Samaan et al. have reported that recurrence rates were lower and survival rates were higher in total thyroidectomized patients [2]. Following total thyroidectomy, I-131 is given for ablation of residual thyroid tissue and treatment of metastatic disease. To achieve a successful ablation and treatment, I-131 should be taken up by residual thyroid and metastatic tumors. The function of cancerous follicular cells is poorer than normal follicular cells. While normal thyroid tissue concentrates 0.5–1.0% of the administered I-131 dose, cancerous cells concentrate 0.01–0.02%.

Papillary cancer (the largest histopathologic group of thyroid cancers), follicular cancer, less than 10% of Hurthle cell variant papillary cancer, and mixed variant medullary cancer show I-131 uptake [3]. Ablation is defined as the radioiodine therapy given for destruction of functional residual thyroid tissue in or out of the thyroid bed. Therapy is the term used for sterilization of residual functional tumoral cells. As the volume of residual thyroid decreases, success of ablation increases. If residual thyroid tissue weighed <2 grams (gr), ablation efficiency was reported as 94%, while this rate may fall as low as 64% in larger residues [4].

The European Association of Nuclear Medicine (EANM) recommends I-131 ablation for all differentiated thyroid cancer patients who have a tumor size >1 cm [5]. For patients with tumor size smaller than <1 cm with no other risk factors like capsular invasion, lymphovascular invasion, lymph node (LN) or distant metastasis, history of radiation exposure, and diffuse sclerosing subtypes, radioiodine ablation is debatable. The American Thyroid Association (ATA) does not recommend radioiodine in low-risk disease [6].

Ablation provides higher thyroglobulin (Tg) sensitivity, treatment of undetectable micrometastatic disease, and a higher survival. Increase in thyroid-stimulating hormone (TSH) levels for ablation helps detection of metastatic disease on the postablative scan. In a prospective study of 25 years of follow-up, it was reported that none of the patients who were totally ablated died of thyroid cancer, but in seven patients in whom ablation failed, the reason of death was thyroid cancer [7]. Thyroid hormone replacement may not be started after surgery to achieve high TSH levels before I-131 therapy performed 4–6 weeks later [8, 9]. However, because euthyroidism augments tissue repair and prevents from postsurgical complications, tetraiodothyronine (T4) replacement therapy is generally started after total thyroidectomy [10].

4. Patient preparation for radioiodine therapy

T4 is stopped before radioiodine therapy and triiodothyronine (T3) can be started instead (25–75 μg/day), making sure that T3 is also withdrawn 2 weeks before I-131 administration [10]. The reason why T3 is given is that T3 has a shorter half-life than T4 (0.8 days versus 7 days) and yields a faster TSH elevation after withdrawal compared to T4. Thus, hypothyroid period is shortened, and potential tumor growth rate stimulated by TSH is decreased.

Low-iodine diet is recommended for 3 weeks before radioiodine treatment, and drugs with stable iodine content should be ceased (**Tables 1** and **2**).

In cases of inadequate TSH elevation (pituitary disease, pituitary insufficiency of the elderly, extensive functioning thyroid cancer metastasis), recombinant human TSH (rhTSH: thyrotropin alpha, Thyrogen®) can be used. 0.9 mg rhTSH is intramuscularly injected for two consecutive days. Twenty-four hours later than the second dose of rhTSH administration, I-131 is given orally. Its safety and efficacy have been found noninferior to endogenous hypothyroidism [11, 12]. There are a few publications mentioned in the use of rhTSH after redifferentiation therapy with retionic acid (13-cis-retinoic acid, isotretinoin) in undifferentiated thyroid cancer to increase radioiodine uptake [13, 14].

Preablative TSH and Tg levels are measured. If TSH is >30 μU/ml, then I-131 can be given [10]. Thyroglobulin is a glycoprotein produced by functioning follicular cells. Detectable Tg after total thyroidectomy is a marker of persistent or recurrent diseases. In subtotal thyroidectomized patients, Tg measurement is not reliable. Thyroglobulin levels should not be used as a single criterion for determining necessity of radioiodine treatment. However, Tg levels

Avoided food
Iodized salt
Milk and derivatives (cheese, yoghurt, ice-cream, etc.)
Seafood
Processed meat products (salami, sausage, etc.)
Packed food (chips, cookies, biscuits, etc.)
Canned vegetables and fruits
Green vegetables (spinach, lettuce, etc.)
Red pepper
Red food dye

Table 1. Avoided food.

Drug or molecule	Recommended withdrawal time
Propylthiouracil, perchlorate, sulfonamides, tapazole, thiocyanate, penicillin, nitrates, antihistamines, and anticoagulants	1 week
Iodine-containing solutions (Lugol's solution, Betadine), antitussives, and vitamin preparates Triiodothyronine (T3)	2 weeks
Tetraiodothyronine (T4)	4–6 weeks
Amiodarone	4–12 weeks
Intravenous contrast agents	1–3 weeks
Oral cholecystographic agents	2–3 weeks

Table 2. Drugs decreasing radioiodine uptake in thyroid cells and recommended withdrawal time.

>5–10 mg/dL point out that there exists an amount of functioning thyroid tissue to be ablated. Conversely, Tg < 1 ng/dL does not exclude radioiodine avid disease either [6].

Patients should be fasting for 2–4 hours before I-131 administration. The aim of fasting is to increase I-131 absorption and decrease risk of vomiting.

5. Radioiodine for ablation

Ablation doses are still a matter of debate. Beierwaltes et al. have reported that 3.7 GBq (100 mCi) I-131 ablates 85% of thyroid remnants [15]. Lower doses of 1.11 GBq (30 mCi) have been shown to be noninferior; however, there are conflicting results [16–19]. There are three approaches for determination of I-131 dose: low dose, fixed high dose, and optimal dose. Low dose refers to 1.11 GBq (30 mCi). If ablation could not be maintained by a single dose, repeated doses can be given by 3–6 months of intervals. Although it depends on local radiation protection rules, hospitalization can be avoided in some regions in the world by dose administration. Lower whole-body and gonadal radiation doses and lower risk of side effects of radioiodine are other advantages. However, if ablation failed, repeated therapies cause long span of hypothyroidism. Stunning is another important disadvantage in secondary ablation doses. Stunning is defined as decrease of radioiodine uptake due to previous I-131 administrations for diagnostic or treatment purposes. Park et al. have reported that diagnostic doses between 111 and 370 MBq (3–10 mCi) I-131 caused stunning in a dose-dependent manner and this effect was overcome by the use of I-123 [20]. I-123 is a good alternative for scanning before I-131 treatment if preablative whole-body scan is necessary, as it gives a lower absorbed dose and provides better image quality and high accuracy [21]. Fixed high doses for ablation are given as 277.5–555 MBq (75–150 mCi). This is an effective and easy method to achieve ablation at a single step, and hypothyroid state is shorter. Nemec et al. have reported that over 85% of the patients ablation was maintained eradicating the need for a second dose [22].

Approach of optimal dose ablation aims to provide ablation of the whole residual thyroid tissue with the lowest radiation burden possible to extrathyroidal tissues [9]. For optimal dose calculation, formulations considering the weight of residual tissue and radioiodine uptake are used:

$$\text{Administered activity}: \frac{\text{Planned dose} \times \text{Gland weight} \times 6.67}{T_{eff} \times \%\,\text{uptake}(24\,\text{hour})} \tag{1}$$

$$\text{Absorbed dose}: \frac{\text{Peak activity of the lesion} \times T_{eff} \times 1.443}{\text{Tissue weight}} \tag{2}$$

T_{eff}: effective half-life

Dose calculation approach may be theoretically reasonable, but it is troublesome to calculate biological half-life by collecting samples of urine and gaita from the patients, and interobserver variabilities in the measurement of residual tissue may cause mistakes. Ablation success rates of fixed high-dose and dose calculation methods are similar. So, fixed high-dose administration is the preferred method with regard to dose calculation.

As I-131 is primarily excreted by urine, dose reduction in renal failure and dialysis should be concerned. Kaptein et al. have reported that in patients who undergo continuous abdominal peritoneal dialysis, radioiodine clearance decreased five times and in order to optimize whole-body and bone marrow dose, radioiodine dose should be reduced by 5 [23]. By dialysis, effective half-life is shortened and tumoral dose is decreased. I-131 administration should be postponed after dialysis. Other situations which cause a change in distribution and increase retention are peritoneal ascites, pleural effusion, and extensive functioning metastasis.

Whole-body I-131 scan should be performed on postablative 2–6 days or after whole-body radiation dose is measured below 370 MBq (10 mCi). This study is important in determination of prognosis, as the absence of detectable metastases decreases risk of recurrence.

6. Adjuvant radioiodine therapy and treatment of metastasis

Postsurgical administration of I-131 provides a significant decline in recurrence rates. This is attributable to adjuvant usage of radioiodine which aims destruction of unknown micrometastasis rather than ablation of residual thyroid [10, 24, 25]. For apparent metastases detected before surgery or in the follow-up, the primary requirement is radioiodine avidity. Fixed high doses are frequently used for treatment of thyroid cancer metastases (**Table 3**).

Another approach in treatment of metastasis is dose calculation according to the upper limits of blood and whole-body dosimetry and quantitative tumor or lesional dosimetry.

Five hundred fifty-five MBq (150 mCi) treats 95% of metastases in the thyroid bed. Upper limit of radioiodine dose for a single administration is determined as 740 MBq (200 mCi), set for a blood radiation dose below 200 rad (200 cGy) (maximum tolerated dose) [9]. In order to provide enough radiation to the tumor, formulations concerning radioiodine uptake value, tumor volume, and effective half-life are used:

$$D(\text{Gy/mCi}): \frac{\%\,\text{uptake}\,(24\,\text{hr}) \times 152 \times T_{eff}}{\text{Tumor mass (gram)}} \tag{3}$$

Metastatic region	Dose GBq (mCi)
Residual thyroid cancer in the thyroid bed	3.7 (100)
Cervical LN metastases	5.55–6.47 (150–175)
Lung metastases	6.47–7.4 (175–200)
Distant metastases	7.4 (200)

Table 3. Doses used in the treatment of functioning thyroid cancer metastasis.

For lymph node metastases, surgery is the first treatment to try, especially in bulky disease. Small LN metastases with adequate radioiodine uptake can be treated with I-131.

Adjunctive radioiodine therapy after surgery is generally recommended. Published in a retrospective series is that, a delay in radioiodine therapy for 6 months or more caused disease progression, and survival rates were decreased [26].

Cervical lymph node involvement doesn't increase mortality but morbidity. The lymph node is common especially in papillary carcinoma, and its incidence has been reported 48 and 17% below and over age 40 [27]. Recurrence rates are twice as much in nodal metastatic disease [10]. It has been proved that recurrent metastases decrease by treatment of metastatic lymph nodes by I-131 [28].

Distant metastasis significantly reduces survival rates. Mortality rates are higher in brain and skeletal metastasis. In a series, distant metastasis was detected in 19% of the patients who received radioiodine treatment. Of these, 44% were to lungs, 31% to mediastinum, and 23% to the skeletal system [29]. Pulmonary metastasis is seen in 2–12% of the cases, and its frequency is less in patients who had undergone total thyroidectomy and radioiodine therapy [28, 30].

Pulmonary metastasis occurs by lymphogen, whereas skeletal metastasis occurs by microinvasion and hematogen way. The fact that there is a correlation between cervical lymph node and pulmonary metastasis and a reverse correlation between nodal and skeletal metastasis supports this opinion. Skeletal metastasis has a worse prognosis than lung metastasis. Skeletal metastasis is seen five times more frequent in follicular carcinoma patients than in papillary carcinoma patients and in the elderly. The cranium, vertebral column, and costae are generally involved [22].

3.7–7.4 GBq (100–200 mCi) I-131 is recommended to be administered by 6–12 months of intervals. Therapy should be continued till all radioiodine avid lesions are ablated or an intolerable complication is likely to arise. For iodine avid disease, there is no upper limit for cumulative dose. However, due to high complication risks, doses over 22.2 GBq (600 mCi) should be evaluated on a patient basis. If complete response can't be achieved but disease stays stable, then intervals between doses can be extended, or therapy can be stopped with close monitoring [5].

7. Differentiated thyroid carcinoma derived from ectopic tissue

Sublingual area is the most common place for ectopic thyroid development. Insufficient T4 production in ectopic tissue may cause TSH elevation and thus hyperplasia by stimulation. Long-term and intense TSH stimulation is blamed for carcinoma development in these cases. Thyroglossal canal originated papillary carcinoma may have an invasive character in 10% of the cases [31]. In 3% of the cases, ectopic thyroid tissue is found in ovarian teratoma (struma ovarii). Low-grade malignant tumor may arise from struma ovarii (5–20%), and some may metastasize [32]. Although management approaches are still uncertain, treatment of cancer of an aberrant thyroid tissue is the excision of the tumor followed by radioiodine therapy.

8. Contraindications

Absolute contraindications are pregnancy and nursing. If I-131 administration is essential, then nursing should be stopped [33, 34]. I-131 passes through the placenta and concentrates in fetal thyroid (<12 weeks). This causes serious hypothyroidism. Maternal bladder activity also causes fetal irradiation. Pregnancy should be avoided for 6–12 weeks after radioiodine therapy. Other relative contraindications for I-131 are bone marrow depression, pulmonary, salivary gland and renal function interruption, possibility of severe edema, and compression symptoms in brain metastasis [5].

9. Complications

There are acute (first 3 months) and chronic (later than 3 months) complications of radioiodine therapy. Acute complications are sialadenitis (most frequent), radiation parotitis and thyroiditis, metallic taste, gastrointestinal symptoms like nausea and vomiting due to radiation gastritis, transient bone marrow depression (anemia in 36% of the patients, leukopenia 10%, thrombocytopenia 3%), radiation pneumonitis and pulmonary fibrosis, radiation cystitis, transient amenorrhea (secondary to pituitary-gonadal hormonal axis), decreased testicular function or fertilization, cerebral edema or spinal compression in metastatic cases, keratoconjunctivitis, and decreased lacrimal function [35]. Chronic complications include secondary malignancies most frequently leukemia, myeloid leukemia, less frequently bladder cancer, salivary gland neoplasia, hypo- and hyperparathyroidism, and hypothyroidism [36–38].

10. Radioiodine therapy of pediatric differentiated thyroid cancer

Prognostic factors in differentiated thyroid cancer of the thyroid are not very well known because it is a relatively rare entity (3–4%) compared to thyroid cancer of the adults. In long-term follow-up, survival rates are found to be high despite increased rates of local recurrences and distant metastasis. Neck and pulmonary metastases concentrate and respond to radioiodine well [10]. Aggressive surgery followed by radioiodine is generally the preferred treatment option [39]. Radioiodine decreases recurrence in patients with known residual disease [40]. Disease-free survival rates are shown to be improved by radioiodine ablation without any significant increase in the risk of secondary malignancies [41]. I-131 treatment is recommended in radioiodine avid unresectable locoregional or distant metastasis [42].

Author details

Derya Cayir* and Mine Araz

*Address all correspondence to: drderyaors@hotmail.com

Nuclear Medicine Department, Dışkapı Yıldırım Beyazıt Training and Research Hospital, Ankara, Turkey

References

[1] Schlumberger MJ. Papillary and follicular thyroid carcinoma. N Engl J Med. 1998:**29**; 338(5):297-306.

[2] Samaan NA, Schultz PN, Hickey RC, Goepfert H, Haynie TP, Johnston DA, Ordonez NG. The results of various modalities of treatment of well differentiated thyroid carcinomas: A retrospective review of 1599 patients. Journal of Clinical Endocrinology and Metabolism. 1992;**75**:714-720

[3] Daniels GH. Radioiodine and thyroid cancer: Some questions, controversies, and considerations. Endocrine Practice. 2001;**7**:320-323

[4] Ross DS. Subclinical hypothyroidism. In: Braverman LE, Utiger RD, editors. Werner and Ingbar's The Thyroid, a Fundamental and Clinical Text. 7th ed. Philadelphia-New York: JP Lippincott-Raven Publishers; 1996. pp. 1010-1015

[5] Luster M, Clarke SE, Dietlein M, Lassmann M, Lind P, Oyen WJ, Tennvall J, Bombardieri E, European Association of Nuclear Medicine (EANM). Guidelines for radioiodine therapy of differentiated thyroid cancer. European Journal of Nuclear Medicine and Molecular Imaging. 2008;**35**:1941-1959

[6] Haugen BR, Alexander EK, Bible KC, Doherty GM, Mandel SJ, Nikiforov YE, Pacini F, Randolph GW, Sawka AM, Schlumberger M, Schuff KG, Sherman SI, Sosa JA, Steward DL, Tuttle RM, Wartofsky L. 2015 American Thyroid Association management guidelines for adult patients with thyroid nodules and differentiated thyroid cancer: The American Thyroid Association guidelines task force on thyroid nodules and differentiated thyroid cancer. Thyroid. 2016;**26**:1-133

[7] Krishnamurthy GT, Blahd WH. Radioiodine I-131 therapy in the management of thyroid cancer. A prospective study. Cancer. 1977;**40**:195-202

[8] Hurley JR, Becker DV. The use of radioiodine in the management of thyroid cancer. In: Freeman LM, Weissman HS, (eds). Nuclear Medicine Annual. New York: Raven Press; 1983. pp. 329-384

[9] Beierwaltes WH. The treatment of thyroid carcinoma with radioactive iodine. Seminars in Nuclear Medicine. 1978;**8**:79-94

[10] Harbert JC. Radioiodine therapy of differentiated thyroid carcinoma. In: Harbert JC, Eckelman WC, Neumann RD, (eds). Nuclear Medicine: Diagnostic and Therapy. 5th ed. New York: Thieme Medical Publishers; 1996. pp. 945-1019

[11] Haugen BR, Pacini F, Reiners C, Schlumberger M, Ladenson PW, Sherman SI, et al. A comparison of recombinant human thyrotropin and thyroid hormone withdrawal for the detection of thyroid remnant or cancer. Journal of Clinical Endocrinology and Metabolism. 1999;**84**:3877-3885

[12] Jarzab B, Handkiewicz-Junak D, Roskosz J, Puch Z, Wygoda Z, et al. Recombinant human TSH-aided radioiodine treatment of advanced differentiated thyroid carcinoma: A single-centre study of 54 patients. European Journal of Nuclear Medicine. 2003;**30**:1077-1086

[13] Schmutzler C, Kohrle J. Retinoic acid redifferentiation therapy for thyroid cancer. Thyroid. 2000;**10**:393-406

[14] Boerner AR, Petrich T, Weckesser M, Langen KJ, Knapp WH. Monitoring isotretinoin therapy in thyroid cancer using 18F-FDG PET. European Journal of Nuclear Medicine. 2002;**29**:231-236

[15] Beierwaltes WH, Rabbani R, Dmuchowski C, Lloyd RV, Eyre P, Mallette S. An analysis of "ablation of thyroid remnants" with I-131 in 511 patients from 1947-1984: Experience at University of Michigan. Journal of Nuclear Medicine. 1984;**25**:1287-1293

[16] Mallick U, Harmer C, Yap B, Wadsley J, Clarke S, Moss L, Nicol A, Clark PM, Farnell K, McCready R, Smellie J, Franklyn JA, John R, Nutting CM, Newbold K, Lemon C, Gerrard G, Abdel-Hamid A, Hardman J, Macias E, Roques T, Whitaker S, Vijayan R, Alvarez P, Beare S, Forsyth S, Kadalayil L, Hackshaw A. Ablation with low-dose radioiodine and thyrotropin alfa in thyroid cancer. The New England Journal of Medicine. 2012;**366**:1674-1685

[17] Kuni CC, Kleingensmith WC 3rd. Failure of low doses of I-131 to ablate residual thyroid tissue following surgery of thyroid cancer. Radiology. 1980;**137**:773-774

[18] DeGroot LJ, Reilly M. Comparison of 30 and 50 mCi doses of iodine-131 for thyroid ablation. Annals of Internal Medicine. 1982;**96**:51-53

[19] Johansen K, Woodhouse NJ, Odugbesan O. Comparison of 1073 MBq and 3700 MBq iodine-131 in postoperative ablation of residual thyroid tissue in patients with differentiated thyroid cancer. Journal of Nuclear Medicine. 1991;**32**:252-254

[20] Park HM, Perkins OW, Edmondson JW, Schnute RB, Manatunga A. Influence of diagnostic radioiodines on the uptake of ablative dose of iodine-131. Thyroid. 1994;**4**:49-54

[21] Park HM, Park YH, Zhou XZ. Detection of thyroid remnant metastases without stunning: An ongoing dilemma. The diagnostic accuracy of 123I and 131I as scanning agents and their effect on the outcome of radioablation therapy. Thyroid. 1997;**7**:277-280

[22] Nemec J, Röhling S, Zamrazil V, Pohunková D. Comparison of the distribution of diagnostic and thyroablative I-131 in the evaluation of differentiated thyroid cancers. Journal of Nuclear Medicine. 1979;**20**:92-97

[23] Kaptein M, Levenson H, Siegel ME, Gadallah M, Akmal M. Radioiodine dosimetry in patients with end-stage renal disease receiving continuous ambulatory peritoneal dialysis therapy. Journal of Clinical and Endocrinology Metabolism. 2000;**85**:3058-3064

[24] Waxman A, Ramanna L, Chapman D, Chapman M, Brachman D, Tanasescu D, Berman B, Catz, Braunstein G. The significance of I-131 scan dose in patients with thyroid cancer. Determination of ablation: Concise communication. Journal of Nuclear Medicine. 1981;**22**:861-865

[25] Němec J, Zamrazil V, Pohunková D, Zeman V, Röhling S. Mode spread of thyroid cancer. Oncology. 1979;**36**:232-235

[26] Higashi T, Nishii R, Yamada S, Nakamoto Y, Ishizu K, Kawase S, Togashi K, Itasaka S, Hiraoka M, Misaki T, Konishi J. Delayed initial radioactive iodine therapy resulted in poor survival in patients with metastatic differentiated thyroid carcinoma: A retrospective statistical analysis of 198 cases. Journal of Nuclear Medicine. 2011;**52**:683-689

[27] Schlumberger M, Fragu P, Gardet P, Lumbroso J, Violot D, Parmentier C. A new immunoradiometric assay (IRMA) system for thyroglobulin measurement in the follow-up of thyroid cancer patients. European Journal of Nuclear Medicine. 1991;**18**:153-157

[28] Mazzaferri EL, Young RL. Papillary thyroid carcinoma: A 10 year follow-up report of the impact of therapy in 576 patients. American Journal of Medicine. 1981;**70**:511-518

[29] Beierwaltes WH, Nishiyama RH, Thompson NW, et al. Survival time and 'cure' in papillary and follicular thyroid carcinoma with distant metastases: Statistics following University of Michigan therapy. Journal of Nuclear Medicine. 1982;**23**:561-580

[30] Young RL, Mazzaferri EL, Rahe AJ, Dorfman SG. Pure follicular thyroid carcinoma: Impact of therapy in 214 patients. Journal of Nuclear Medicine. 1980;**21**:733-737

[31] DeGroot LJ, Larsen PR, Refetoff S, Stanbury JB. The Thyroid and Its Diseases. 5th ed. New York: John Wiley & Sons; 1984. p. 633

[32] Fox H, Langley FA. Tumors of the Ovary. England: Heinemann Medical Books; 1976. p. 236

[33] Robinson PS, Barker P, Campbell A, Henson P, Surveyor I, Young PR. Iodine-131 in breast milk following therapy for thyroid carcinoma. Journal of Nuclear Medicine. 1994;**35**:1797-1801

[34] Mountfort PJ. Restrictions following iodine-131 treatment: A time for charge or more data required?. European Journal of Nuclear Medicine. 1994;**22**:903-905

[35] Haynie TP, Beierwaltes WH. Hematologic changes observed following I-131 therapy for thyroid carcinoma. Journal of Nuclear Medicine. 1963;**4**:85-91

[36] Brincker H, Hansen HS, Andersen AP. Induction of leukaemia by I-131 treatment of thyroid carcinoma. British Journal of Cancer. 1973;**28**:232-237

[37] Refetoff S, Harrison J, Kavanfilski BT, Kaplan EL, De Groot LJ, Bekerman C. Continuing occurrence of thyroid carcinoma after irradiation to the neck in infancy and childhood. The New England Journal of Medicine. 1975;**292**:171-175

[38] Beierwaltes WH. The treatment of hyperthyroidism with iodine-131. Seminars in Nuclear Medicine. 1978;**8**:95-103

[39] Jarzab B, Junak DH, Wloch J, Kalemba B, Roskosz J, Kukulska A, Puch Z. Multivariate analysis of prognostic factors for differentiated thyroid carcinoma in children. European Journal of Nuclear Medicine. 2000;**27**:833-841

[40] Chow SM, Law SC, Mendenhall WM, Au SK, Yau S, Mang O, Lau WH. Differentiated thyroid carcinoma in childhood and adolescence-clinical course and role of radioiodine. Pediatric Blood Cancer. 2004;**42**:176-183

[41] Jarzab B, Handkiewicz-Junak D, Wloch J. Juvenile differentiated thyroid carcinoma and the role of radioiodine in its treatment: A qualitative review. Endocrine Related Cancer. 2005;**12**:773-803

[42] Francis GL, Waguespack SG, Bauer AJ, Angelos P, Benvenga S, Cerutti JM, Dinauer CA, Hamilton J, Hay ID, Luster M, Parisi MT, Rachmiel M, Thompson GB, Yamashita S. American Thyroid Association Guidelines Task Force. Management guidelines for children with thyroid nodules and differentiated thyroid cancer. Thyroid. 2015 Jul;**25** (7):716-759

Section 2

Other Radionuclide Treatments

Chapter 3

I-131 Metaiodobenzylguanidine Therapy of Neuroectodermal Tumors

Mine Araz and Derya Çayır

Additional information is available at the end of the chapter

http://dx.doi.org/10.5772/intechopen.68573

Abstract

I-131 metaiodobenzylguanidine (MIBG) is a noradrenaline analogue and acts as an adrenergic neuron blocker. It is commonly used in the radionuclide treatment of neuroectodermal-derived tumors (Stage III–IV neuroblastoma, inoperable pheochromocytoma, paraganglioma and carcinoid tumor, metastatic or recurrent medullary thyroid cancer). These are rare tumors and clinical data about therapeutic options accumulate slowly. I-131 MIBG has a well-known role in the salvage therapy of these tumors; however, recent data suggest that it may also be beneficial to use as the first-line method. Here, we define characteristics of the radiopharmaceutical, mention cautions during administration and discuss clinical applications of I-131 MIBG therapy of the neuroectodermal tumors.

Keywords: iodobenzylguanidine, neuroectodermal tumors, therapeutics, neoplasms, radiation

1. Introduction

Metaiodobenzylguanidine (MIBG, Iobenguane) is an aralkylguanidine analogue, composed of bretylium and guanethidine (an adrenergic neuron blocker). It acts as a noradrenaline analogue and is taken up by adrenergic sympathetically innervated tissues. Neural crest originated tumors, which are derived from sympathetic nervous system, are therefore suitable for scintigraphic imaging and targeted therapy with radioiodine-labeled MIBG. I-131-labeled MIBG is the compound used for therapy in neuroectodermal tumors. These tumors have a very low incidence, and thus clinical experience in therapy with I-131 MIBG is limited to specific reference centers. This chapter aims to give information about the physical characteristics of I-131 MIBG, uptake mechanisms of the radiocompound in the tumoral tissue, indications and contraindications for I-131 MIBG therapy, specifications for the facility where the therapy will be performed, patient preparation and administration of I-131 MIBG, follow-up and precautions on possible side effects and make an overview on the clinical studies about I-131 MIBG therapy.

2. Radiopharmaceutical

I-131 MIBG is a "theranostic," the term that stands for the agents used for both diagnostic and therapeutic approach [1]. Physical properties of I-131 bring in this advantage. I-131 has a gamma ray at 364 keV and a mean beta emission of 606 keV. Beta particular emission causes cell death, and gamma rays are used for scintigraphic imaging. A half-life of 8.02 days provides enough time for labeling and shipping [2].

Metaiodobenzylguanidine (MIBG) is a synthetic analogue of norepinephrine and an aralkylguanidine, a combination of benzyl group of bretylium and guanidine group of guanethidine [3]. The reason why MIBG is the preferred pharmaceutical among other aralkylguanidines is that it shows the lowest liver uptake, the best in vivo stability, and thus, lowest amount of free radioiodine is trapped by thyroid tissue. In a study by Wieland et al., 100 μCi I-125-labeled iodobenzylguanidine isomers (para, ortho and meta) were intravenously administered to 41 mongrel dogs separately. Following injections, tissue distribution of each isomer in a given time was detected by obtaining samples from 18 different tissues. They found out that meta and para isomers were taken up by adrenal medulla starting from 2 h of injection and lasted till 8 days. Despite adrenal medulla is surrounded by liver, an organ with metabolic activity and adrenergic innervation, even on the measurements, performed on 5 days of injection, the ratio of adrenal medulla counts/liver counts was calculated as high as 1000. In addition to adrenal medulla, high amount of radiopharmaceutical uptake was detected in thyroid. However, detailed analysis of thyroid tissue measurements revealed that meta-isomer was more resistant to in vivo deiodination [4].

I-131 MIBG is rapidly cleared from bloodstream following intravenous administration and taken up by adrenergically innervated tissues like adrenal medulla, heart and salivary glands. In the first hour, heart and lungs are major apparent organs. Maximal uptake in the tumoral tissue occurs 24–96 h later. The major route of elimination of the radiopharmaceutical is glomerular filtration. In subject with normal renal function, 50% of the administered activity was shown to be excreted unchanged via urine in 24 h and 90% is eliminated by the kidneys in 4 days. A very small amount of I-131 MIBG is metabolized in vivo (<10%). End products are m-iodohippuric acid, m-iodobenzoic acid, 4-hydroxy-3-iodobenzylguanidine and free radioiodine [5, 6].

Norepinephrine (NE) is synthesized by dopamine-hydroxylase from dopamine (DA) in presynaptic neurons of adrenal medulla, carried by the vesicles and secreted to the synaptic gap. NE then binds to pre- and postsynaptic adrenergic receptors in the synaptic gap. NE is reuptaken by the pre- and postsynaptic cells through NE transporters (NETs) and stored in the vesicles. This reuptake process is called "specific neuronal uptake 1" and is Na and energy (ATP) dependant. Ligand affinity is high, whereas saturability is low. It is sensitive to heat and ouabaine, Na+/K+/ATP'ase inhibitor. MIBG, the Ne analogue, acts similar to NE. As the molecular structure remains unchanged, I-131-labeled MIBG is also taken up by the NET expressing cells (mainly derived from the neural crest), using NETs. However, this specific mechanism of uptake is not the only uptake mechanism of I-131 MIBG uptake in cellular level. The second mechanism is nonspecific passive diffusion, which takes place in all cell types. Specific neuronal uptake is 50 times more effective than passive diffusion [4, 7, 8]. After internalized in the cell, I-131 MIBG is taken up by vesicular monoamine transporters (VMAT 1 and 2) and stored in neurosecretory granules [9].

3. Indications

Although any tumor capable of I-131 uptake on pretherapy I-131 MIBG scan may have a chance to be treated with I-131 MIBG, I-131 MIBG has a well-established place only in therapy regimen of some common neuroendocrine tumors: Stage III–IV neuroblastoma (NB), inoperable pheochromocytoma, paraganglioma and carcinoid tumor, metastatic or recurrent medullary thyroid cancer [10]. To decide whether a neuroendocrine tumor patient is eligible to I-131 MIBG therapy, I-131 MIBG avidity should be concerned first. This decision can be made either visually (lesions detectable above background activity on I-123 or I-131 MIBG scan) or semiquantitatively (like target/background >2, or >1% of the injected activity taken up by the tumor) [11–16].

4. Contraindications

Absolute contraindications for I-131 MIBG therapy are given as pregnancy and breast feeding. If life expectancy is less than 3 months, therapy is not recommended except for those given for pain palliation. Renal insufficiency is also an undesirable condition for I-131MIBG therapy. Relative contraindications include inconvenient isolation conditions, urinary incontinence, progressive deterioration in renal functions (GFR < 30 ml/min) and myelotoxicity (WBC < 3.0×10^9/l, PLT < 100×10^9/l). Patients susceptible to toxicities should be followed up closely and activity reduction should be concerned [10].

5. Protocol

5.1. Patient preparation

5.1.1. Eligibility for I-131 MIBG therapy

Patients should be evaluated with I-131 or I-123 MIBG scan before therapy to make sure that the tumoral lesions are I-131 MIBG avid [17].

5.1.2. *Thyroid blockade*

Unbound or in vivo radiolyzed free radioiodine is taken up by the thyroid and may cause destruction. Thyroidal uptake should be inhibited by oral stable iodine. Oral iodine (16–130 mg/day) or potassium perchlorate capsules (100–400 m/day) can be used, although iodine capsules are more preferred in pediatric patients because of its better taste. Lugol solution is a simpler alternative, administered 1 drop/kg/day with a maximum of 40 (20 drops twice a day). The treatment should begin 48–24 h before I-131 MIBG administration and continued for 10–15 days after therapy [10].

5.1.3. *Drug interactions*

Various drugs interfere with I-131 MIBG uptake in the target tissue. Drug groups and recommended withdrawal times are presented in **Table 1**. They may inhibit Na-dependent uptake to cell, intracellular vesicular uptake, depletion of I-131 MIBG from the granules, Ca-mediated uptake and some other unproven pathways [10].

Neuroendocrine tumors, especially PHEO and paragangliomas (PGLs), present with hypertension and tachycardia due to secreted catecholamines. Management includes alpha and beta blockers. Discontinuation of these drugs is needed before I-131 MIBG therapy. This causes

Group	Recommended withdrawal time
Antiarrhythmics (amiodaron)	Not practical
Combined alpha-beta blockers (labetolol)	72 h
Adrenergic neuron blockers	48 h
Alpha blockers	15 days
Calcium channel blockers	24–48 h
Inotropic sympathomimetics	24 h
Vasoconstrictor sympathomimetics	24 h
B2 stimulants	24 h
Other adrenoreceptor stimulants (Orciprenaline)	24 h
Systemic and nasal decongestants, cough and cold preparations	24–48 h
Sympathomimetics for glaucoma	48 h
Antipsychotics	24 h–15 days
Sedatizing antihistaminics	24 h
Opioid analgesic drugs	24 h
Tricyclic antidepressants	24–48 h
Tricyclic-related antidepressants	48 h–3 days
CNS stimulants	24 h–5 days

Table 1. Drug groups which may interfere with I-131 MIBG uptake and recommended withdrawal time.

an interruption in symptomatic management. Alpha blocker phenoxybenzamine and beta blocker atenolole do not interfere with I-131 MIBG uptake. Among calcium channel blockers, nifedipine is a safe option, as interference has not been reported [18].

5.2. Dose administration

The radiopharmaceutical administration can be performed either in or outpatient, according to the amount of activity administered and local radiation protection rules. If performed in-patient, dose administration should be performed in an approved nuclear medicine facility with appropriately shielded rooms, radiation safety equipment and capability of management in case of contamination. Dose administration should be supervised by an authorized person, that is, according to the most local commissions, a nuclear medicine specialist [10].

I-131 MIBG is injected intravenously by slow infusion over 1–2 h in a lead shielded infusion set [10, 19, 20]. Possible side effects caused by cold MIBG are aimed to be avoided by slow infusion. It has been stated that I-131 MIBG at high specific activity has a lower potential to cause side effects and thus can be infused in a shorter time period [21].

Vital signs should be closely monitored during and after I-131 MIBG infusion. Short-acting alpha and beta blockers should be kept ready during and after infusion in case sympathetic discharge symptoms occur. I-131 MIBG infusion can be slowed down or stopped if hypertension is unstable [10].

5.3. Determination of activity

Empirical fixed dose, fixed activity per body weight or dosimetrically estimated doses can be given. Single administered activities range between 100 and 300 mCi (3.7–11.2 GBq). Dosimetric calculation is based on dose-limiting side effect, myelotoxicity. Activities delivering 2–4 Gy dose to blood are calculated. Much higher doses than fixed doses can be given by dosimetric approach [22].

In case of repeat administrations, therapy response and toxicities should be taken in consideration to decide which dose to be given. Dose reduction would be appropriate in case of hematologic or renal insufficiency [10]

6. Clinical manifestations

6.1. Neuroblastoma

Neuroblastoma (NB) is the most frequent extracranial tumor of childhood (constituting 8–10% of the pediatric tumors) and presents with metastatic disease in almost half of the cases. Originating from the neural crest, NB can be found anywhere in the sympathetic ganglion chain but mostly in the adrenal gland [23]. Because of the fact that neuroblastomas show high affinity for I-131 MIBG (>90%), I-131 MIBG therapy is of clinical interest for selective internal radiotherapy of NB [10, 24].

Historically, I-131 MIBG was first tried in refractory or relapsed NB patients. Early Phase I dose escalation studies investigated I-131 MIBG as a single agent in the therapy of refractory neuroblastoma. Several dose regimens have been tried by different investigators, yielding a wide range of complete and partial response (CR and PR): 0–66% [25–35]. Weight-based dose arrangement is now well established. 2–6 mCi (74–222 MBq)/kg cause mild hematological side effects but does not provide a high antitumor efficacy either. Significant antitumoral effects start at doses over >6 mCi(222 MBq)/kg [36]. However, the degree of bone marrow depression increases by rising doses, and a new approach was developed combining higher effective doses with prior cryopreservation of stem cells and bone marrow transplantation following I-131 MIBG therapy. Greater than 12 mCi (444 MBq)/kg is the settled limit for stem cell rescue [37]. Doses above 15 mCi (555 MBq)/kg are now used for myeloablation either with or without myeloablative chemotherapies [36]. Matthay et al. have published a large trial of I-131 MIBG monotherapy in refractory or relapsed NB. The vast majority of the patient group received 18 mCi (666 MBq)/kg I-131 MIBG, whereas others were given 12 mCi (444 MBq)/kg. Overall CR and PR rates were found 36%. However, investigators also revealed that age, site of disease involvement, previously received therapies and time between first diagnosis and first I-131 MIBG dose are important in prediction of treatment success. Response rates were 55 and 40% above and below age 12, respectively. Soft tissue, skeletal and bone marrow involvement responded in 50, 45 and 26%, respectively. Event-free survival rate was found 18%, and 2-year overall survival was 29%. Together with hematologic toxicity, to a lesser extent, other side effects such as hepatic, pulmonary and infectious toxicities and febrile neutropenia were also reported in this study [38].

I-131 MIBG monotherapy is also combined with myeloablative chemotherapies to be used in higher doses with stem cell rescue. A leading study by Yanik et al. suggested that carboplatine-etoposide-melphelan in combination with I-131 MIBG therapy administered in 12 mCi (444 MBq)/kg doses in 12 patients. Therapy was well tolerated and 5/8 patients with metastatic disease showed complete and 2/8 showed partial response [39]. In a larger cohort group, 3-year event-free survival and overall survival rates were found 38 and 20% in patients who had a PR to induction therapy and 20 and 62% in patients who had a progressive disease [40]. It was also reported that I-131 MIBG was not detrimental to hematologic recovery after stem cell transplantation [41].

In 2000s, in relapsed or refractory NB patients, tandem doses of I-131 MIBG infusions were tried. The best therapy responses were achieved after initial dose administration and response rates decreased by repeat infusions. That was also true for patients who have already received myeloablative doses of I-131 MIBG (>18 Mci(666 MBq)/kg) [42–44]. Although well tolerated, overall clinical response rates in a meta-analysis were reported as 30%, even in tandem infusions [45]. This leads the investigators to seek for other strategies to increase the efficacy of I-131 MIBG therapy. NET expression increase would be very beneficial to increase I-131 MIBG uptake by the tumor cells. Among the chemotherapeuticals, cisplatin and topotecan are agents of choice to augment NET expression. While response rates were ameliorated, side effects were not significantly aggravated [46, 47]. In a study of refractory NB patients who received 200 mCi (7.4 GBq) I-131 MIBG in combination with cisplatin, cyclophosphamide (plus etoposide and vincristine or not), an overall response rate of 75% was achieved [46].

Promising results experienced over years with I-131 MIBG therapy have lead to a new approach, usage of I-131 MIBG in the front-line as a part of the induction therapy for patients who do not have a relapsed or refractory tumor yet. Investigators have found that I-131 MIBG avid tumors, which are not exposed to chemo-radiotherapies yet, are more responsive to I-131 MIBG therapy given at the early steps of the therapy algorithm. In the preoperative period, I-131 MIBG therapy performed at diagnosis was reported to lead to a response rate of over 70%, which is obviously higher than the rates obtained after conventional therapies [48]. De Kraker et al. proposed three major arguments: First, if performed before surgery, I-131 MIBG reduced the volume of the primary and metastatic tumors. Second, overlapping toxic situations confronted with chemotherapy in combination therapies are avoided. Finally, cross-fire effect achieved at the first-line therapy, the ability of the radiation dose given to a tumor cell also causes death of the neighboring cells. The authors published the largest study in this field with 44 high-risk patients who received two cycles of I-131 MIBG as an induction therapy and received a response rate of 73% [49]. Bleeker et al. have also reported that together with high success rates, side effects were also lower [50]. Combination of I-131 MIBG with chemotherapeuticals did not cause a significant increase in side effects [50, 51].

Pain palliation with I-131 MIBG is another secondary benefit reported commonly in NB [31]. Low dose (5 mCi (185 MBq)/kg) I-131 MIBG has also been suggested as an effective means for pain palliation in metastatic disease [52].

6.2. Pheochromocytoma and paraganglioma

Paragangliomas (PGL) arise from sympathetic chromaffin tissue (adrenal or extraadrenal) and parasympathetic ganglions of the head and neck. Pheochromocytomas (PCC), which originate from the adrenal medulla, constitute 80% of all paragangliomas (PG) [53, 54]. Most PGLs are benign, while about 10% of PCCs and 10–20% of extraadrenal non-head and neck PGLs may undergo malignant degeneration [55]. Malignant disease refers to existence of metastatic lesions where neuroendocrine tissue is not expected to exist [56–58]. In malignant PCC/PGL, malignant disease has a bad prognosis and together with palliative therapy, I-131 MIBG has been tried [59, 60].

I-131 MIBG was first tried by Sission et al. on MIBG avid PCC patients. Fractionated doses of a total of 373–484 mCi (13.8–17.9 GBq) I-131 MIBG was given to five patients and two patients responded partially. Hormone secretion was decreased and tumor volume declined by more than 50% in these patients [37, 61]. Many other series with larger number of patients came afterwards. However, it is hard to make a final conclusion about the effectiveness of I-131 MIBG therapy on PCC/PGLs because these studies differed in many ways. First of all, as PCC/PGLs are relatively rare tumors, study populations were small and heterogenous in many studies. Patient selection criteria for I-131 MIBG therapy varied. Some administered I-131 MIBG therapy only in progressive cases, while in some studies patients with stable disease were also included. In stable cases, stability may not be totally attributable to the effectiveness of I-131 MIBG therapy, as these patients may already have stayed progress free even if no additional therapies were given. The amount of activity, dose fractionation, time elapsed between two therapy sessions, tumor response and hormonal response evaluation criteria were all set differently in these cohorts. Moreover, PCC and PGLs may respond differently to I-131 MIBG therapy, and separate analysis of them could give more accurate and realistic results.

In the literature, generally low (64–200 mCi) (2.368–7.4 GBq), intermediate (200–500 mCi) (7.4–18.5 MBq) and high (1.2–1.8 mCi) (444–666 GBq) doses of I-131 MIBG with stem cell support have been tried. Low and intermediate doses were chosen in order to be able to give repeat doses and thus decrease toxicities. Tandem doses resulted in cumulative doses as high as 2.3 Ci (85.1 MBq), but usually in a range of 500–1000 mCi (18.5–37 MBq). A review analyzing the results of repeat low dose I-131 MIBG, CR, PR, SD and PD rates were found 4, 26, 50 and 13%, respectively. Objective hormonal response was obtained completely in 13% and partially in 32%. Symptomatic relief due to hormonal excess was maintained in 76% of the patients [62]. Comparison of three methodologies was reported in 33 patients. Median survival was 4.7 years for patients responding to I-131 MIBG therapy and 1.7 years for nonresponders. Patients who received high doses (>500 mCi) (>18.5 MBq) had a higher survival rate than the low dose group (3.8 versus 2.6 years) [63]. A recent meta-analysis by Hulsteijn et al. aimed to present effectiveness of I-131 MIBG therapy in malignant PCC/PGL. If effects on tumor volume are considered, pooled proportions of CR, PR and SD were found to be 0.03, 0.27 and 0.52, respectively. Hormonal response rates were 0.11, 0.4 and 0.21, respectively. Five-year survival rates ranged between 45 and 64% and PFSs were 23.1–28.5 months. A separate analysis revealed better hormonal response in PGL than PCC [64].

6.3. Others

The use of I-131 MIBG in carcinoid tumors and medullary thyroid carcinoma has been reported in relapse or refractory cases. Certain eligibility criterion is of course I-131 MIBG avidity proven by I-123 MIBG scan. I-131 MIBG therapy in these patients is rather palliative and aims to increase quality of life. Medullary thyroid carcinoma is rare and only about 34% of medullary thyroid cancer patients have an I-131 MIBG avidity; thus, the experience in this field is quite limited [24, 65–67]. In a study by Safford et al., a relatively wider group of patients with metastatic carcinoid tumor were given 77–1076 mCi (2.849–39.812 GBq) (mean 400 mCi) (mean 14.8 GBq) I-131 MIBG in 1–3 fractions. Symptomatic relief was gained in about half of the patients (49%). However, only 15% of them showed tumor volume decrease, and no significant effect on survival was reported [68].

7. Toxicity

Early side effects of I-131 MIBG therapy occur in the first hours or days of treatment. Nausea and vomiting are common side effects caused by acute radiation gastritis. Antiemetics are routinely recommended before the infusion starts. Its incidence has been reported between 4 and 40% [20, 69–73]. During I-131 MIBG infusion, catecholamine discharge may cause hypertension and tachycardia in 20% of the patients [11]. Although slow infusion and high specific activity preparations may decrease probability, alpha and beta blockers should be prepared to be used in case of emergency. Acute parotitis can be caused by I-131 MIBG uptake in the salivary glands. Anti-inflammatory agents may help symptomatic relief. Chronic xerostomia has not been reported yet [74].

The most important subacute toxicity is hematotoxicity. Bone marrow is the dose-limiting organ for I-131 MIBG therapy. Because I-131 MIBG binds to platelets, thrombocytopenia is usually more apparent than leucopenia. Hematotoxicity is dose dependent. Doses above 12 mCi(444 MBq)/kg have been shown to cause severe bone marrow toxicity, and in cases of doses exceeding 15 mCi(555 MBq)/kg or repeat doses, stem cell support is required [24, 75, 76].

Late complications of I-131 MIBG include hypothyroidism and secondary malignancies. Hypothyroidism is a result of destruction caused by free radioiodine existing in the product or released after I-131 is metabolized. It is seen months or years after therapy in about 7–12% of the patients [77–81]. This is why thyroid blocking is essential during therapy.

Secondary malignancies such as myelodisplastic syndrome (MDS) and acute myelogenous leukemia (AML) have been reported in about 2–4% of patients [82–84]. As these patients are treated with chemo-radiotherapies in combination with I-131 MIBG, the contribution of I-131 MIBG alone to secondary malignancy development is a matter of debate. Alkylator-based chemotherapeuticals and external radiotherapy are also responsible for mutagenic effects [85].

Other side effects of I-131 MIBG such as pulmonary, cardiac and neurologic complications are rare. However, as liver shows high I-131 MIBG uptake, hepatotoxicity may become clinically evident at high doses. However, this effect is usually transient and aggravated by combination chemo-radiotherapies [81, 86]. Hypogonadism has been reported in higher frequencies with higher I-131 MIBG doses [11, 73, 87].

8. Noncarrier-added I-131 MIBG: an attempt to increase therapy efficiency

I-131 MIBG is synthesized from I-127 MIBG (cold MIBG) by substituting stable iodine by radioiodine [88]. The end product contains I-131 MIBG/I-127 MIBG ratio of 1:2000 [89]. This impurity causes a competition of I-131 and I-127 MIBG for NET and heterogenous tumoral uptake of I-131 MIBG, leaving a considerable amount of tumor cells nonirradiated. Excess MIBG, by the way, can cause symptoms due to sympathetic discharge. Non-carrier added I-131 MIBG was developed both to increase efficiency and to decrease side effects [90]. Noncarrier-added I-131 MIBG will probably be a favorable alternative form after toxicity, and dose escalation studies are completed [91].

Author details

Mine Araz* and Derya Çayır

*Address all correspondence to: minesoylu@yahoo.com

Nuclear Medicine Department, Diskapi Yildirim Beyazit Training and Research Hospital, Ankara, Turkey

References

[1] McCready VR. Radioiodine—The success story of Nuclear Medicine: 75th anniversary of the first use of Iodine-131 in humans. European Journal of Nuclear Medicine and Molecular Imaging. 2017;**44**:179-182

[2] Saha GB. Characteristics of specific radiopharmaceuticals. Fundamentals of Nuclear Pharmacy. 4th ed. New York: Springer Verlag; 1998. pp. 112-147

[3] Vallabhajosula S, Nikolopoulou A. Radioiodinated metaiodobenzylguanidine (MIBG): Radiochemistry, biology, and pharmacology. Seminars in Nuclear Medicine. 2011;**41**: 324-333

[4] Wieland DM, Wu J, Brown LE, et al. Radiolabeled adrenergic neuron-blocking agents: Adrenomedullary imaging with [131I]iodobenzylguanidine. Journal of Nuclear Medicine. 1980;**21**:349-353

[5] Boersma HH, Wensing JW, Kho TL, de Brauw LM, Liem IH, van Kroonenburgh MJ. Transient enhance uptake of ^{123}I-metaiodobenzylguanidine in the contralateral adrenal region after resection of an adrenal pheochromocytoma. The New England Journal of Medicine. 2000;**342**:1450-1451

[6] Mangner TJ, Tobes MC, Wieland DM, et al. Metabolism of meta-I-131-iodobenzyl-guanidine in patients with metastatic pheochromocytoma. Journal of Nuclear Medicine. 1986;**27**:37-44

[7] Wieland DM, Brown LE, Tobes MC, et al: Imaging the primate adrenal medulla with [^{123}I] and [^{131}I] meta-iodobenzylguanidine: Concise communication. Journal of Nuclear Medicine. 1981;**22**:358-364

[8] Wafelman AR, Hoefnagel CA, Maes RA, Beijnen JH. Radioiodinated metaiodobenzylguanidine: A review of its biodistribution and pharmacokinetics, drug interaction, cytotoxicity and dosimetry. European Journal of Nuclear Medicine. 1994;**21**:545-559

[9] Kölby L, Bernhardt P, Levin-Jakobsen AM, Johanson V, Wängberg B, Ahlman H, Forssell-Aronsson E, Nilsson O. Uptake of meta-iodobenzylguanidine in neuroendocrine tumours is mediated by vesicular monoamine transporters. British Journal of Cancer. 2003;**89**(7):1383-1388

[10] Giammarile F, Chiti A, Lassmann M, Brans B, Flux G. EANM guideline: EANM procedure guidelines for ^{131}I-meta-iodobenzylguanidine (^{131}I-mIBG) therapy. European Journal of Nuclear Medicine and Molecular Imaging. 2008;**35**:1039-1047

[11] Gonias S, Goldsby R, Matthay KK, et al. Phase II study of highdose [^{131}I] metaiodobenzylguanidine therapy for patients with metastatic pheochromocytoma and paraganglioma. Journal of Clinical Oncology. 2009;**27**:4162-4168

[12] Pasieka JL, McEwan AJB, Rorstad O. The palliative role of I-131-MIBG and In-111-octreotide therapy in patients with metastatic progressive neuroendocrine neoplasms. Surgery. 2004;**136**:1218-1226

[13] Nguyen C, Faraggi M, Giraudet AL, et al. Long-term efficacy of radionuclide therapy in patients with disseminated neuroendocrine tumors uncontrolled by conventional therapy. Journal of Nuclear Medicine. 2004;**45**:1660-1668

[14] Shapiro B, Sisson JC, Lloyd R, et al. Malignant pheochromocytoma—Clinical, biochemical and scintigraphic characterization. Clinical Endocrinology. 1984;**20**:189-203

[15] Taal BG, Hoefnagel CA, Valdes-Olmos RA, et al. Palliative effect of metaiodobenzylguanidine in metastatic carcinoid tumors. Journal of Clinical Oncology. 1996;**14**:1829-1838

[16] Pathirana AA, Vinjamuri S, Byrne C, et al. I-131-MIBG radionuclide therapy is safe and cost-effective in the control of symptoms of the carcinoid syndrome. European Journal of Surgical Oncology. 2001;**27**:404-408

[17] Vaidyanathan G. Meta-iodobenzylguanidine and analogues: Chemistry and biology. The Quarterly Journal of Nuclear Medicine and Molecular Imaging. 2008;**52**:351-368

[18] Blake GM, Lewington VJ, Fleming JS, et al. Modification by nifedipine of I-131-meta-iodobenzylguanidine kinetics in malignant pheochromocytoma. European Journal of Nuclear Medicine. 1988;**14**:345-348

[19] Schlumberger M, Gicquel C, Lumbroso J, et al. Malignant pheochromocytoma-Clinical, biological, histologic and therapeutic data in a series of 20 patients with distant metastases. Journal of Endocrinological Investigation. 1992;**15**:631-642

[20] Shapiro B, Sisson JC, Wieland DM, et al. Radiopharmaceutical therapy of malignant pheochromocytoma with I-131 metaiodobenzylguanidine: Results from ten years of experience. Journal of Nuclear Biology and Medicine. 1991;**35**:269-276

[21] Coleman RE, Stubbs JB, Barrett JA, et al. Radiation dosimetry, pharmacokinetics, and safety of ultratrace (TM) iobenguane I-131 in patients with malignant pheochromocytoma/paraganglioma or meta-static carcinoid. Cancer Biotherapy and Radiopharmaceuticals. 2009;**24**:469-475

[22] Carrasquillo JA, Pandit-Taskar N, Chen CC. I-131 metaiodobenzylguanidine therapy of pheochromocytoma and paraganglioma. Seminars in Nuclear Medicine. 2016;**46**:203-214

[23] Luksch R, Castellani MR, Collini P, De Bernardi B, Conte M, Gambini C, Gandola L, Garaventa A, Biasoni D, Podda M, Sementa AR, Gatta G, Tonini GP. Neuroblastoma (Peripheral neuroblastic tumours). Critical Reviews in Oncology/Hematology. 2016;**107**: 163-181

[24] Sisson JC, Yanik GA. Theranostics: Evolution of the radiopharmaceutical. Seminars in Nuclear Medicine. 2012;**42**:171-184

[25] Hutchinson RJ, Sisson JC, Miser JS, et al. Long-term results of [131I] metaiodobenzylguanidine treatment of refractory advanced neuroblastoma. Journal of Nuclear Biology and Medicine. 1991;**35**:237-240

[26] Hutchinson RJ, Sisson JC, Shapiro B, et al. 131-I metaiodobenzylguanidine treatment in patients with refractory advanced neuroblastoma. American Journal of Clinical Oncology. 1992;**15**:226-232

[27] Lashford LS, Lewis IJ, Fielding SL, et al. Phase I/II study of iodine 131 metaiodobenzylguanidine in chemoresistant neuroblastoma. A United Kingdom children's cancer study group investigation. Journal of Clinical Oncology. 1992;**10**:1889-1896

[28] Matthay KK, Huberty JP, Hattner RS, et al. Efficacy and safety of [^{131}I] metaiodobenzylguanidine therapy for patients with refractory neuroblastoma. Journal of Nuclear Biology and Medicine. 1991;**35**:244-247

[29] Klingebiel T, Feine U, Treuner J, et al. Treatment of neuroblastoma with [^{131}I] metaiodobenzylguanidine: Long-term results in 25 patients. Journal of Nuclear Biology and Medicine. 1991;**35**:216-219

[30] Trancone L, Rufini V, Riccardi R, et al. The use of [^{131}I] metaiodobenzylguanidine in the treatment of neuroblastoma after conventional therapy. Journal of Nuclear Biology and Medicine. 1991;**35**:232-236

[31] Kang TI, Brophy P, Hickson M, et al. Targeted radiotherapy with submyeloablative doses of ^{131}I MIBG is effective for disease palliation in highly refractory neuroblastoma. Journal of Pediatric Hematology/Oncology. 2003;**25**:769-773

[32] Claudiani F, Garaventa A, Bertolazzi L, et al. [^{131}I] metaiodobenzylguanidine therapy in advanced neuroblastoma. Journal of Nuclear Biology and Medicine. 1991;**35**:224-227

[33] Garaventa A, Bellgamba O, Lo Piccolo MS, et al. ^{131}I-metaiodobenzylguanidine (^{131}I-MIBG) therapy for residual neuroblastoma. A mono-institutional experience with 43 patients. British Journal of Cancer. 1999;**81**:1378-1384

[34] Hoefnagel CA, Voute PA, De Kraker J, et al. [^{131}I] metaiodobenzylguanidine therapy after conventional therapy for neuroblastoma. Journal of Nuclear Biology and Medicine. 1991;**35**:202-206

[35] Lumbroso J, Hartmann O, Schlumberger M. Therapeutic use of [^{131}I] metaiodobenzylguanidine in neuroblastoma. A phase II study in 26 patients. Societe Francaised'oncologie pediatrique and nuclear medicine co-investigators. Journal of Nuclear Biology and Medicine. 1991;**35**:220-223

[36] Parisi MT, Eslamy H, Park JR, Shulkin BL, Yanik GA. ^{131}I-metaiodobenzylguanidine theranostics in neuroblastoma: Historical perspectives; practical applications. Seminars in Nuclear Medicine. 2016;**46**:184-202

[37] Matthay KK, De Santes K, Hasegawa B, et al. Phase I dose escalation of ^{131}I-metaiodobenzylguanidine with autologous bone marrow support in refractory neuroblastoma. Journal of Clinical Oncology. 1998;**16**:229-236

[38] Matthay KK, Yanik G, Messina J, et al. Phase II study on the effect of disease sites, age, and prior therapy on response to iodine-131-metaiodobenzylguanidine therapy in refractory neuroblastoma. Journal of Clinical Oncology. 2007;**25**:105410-105460

[39] Yanik GA, Levine JE, Matthay KK. Pilot study of iodine-131-metaiodobenzylguanidine in combination with myeloablative chemotherapy and autologous stem-cell support for the treatment of neuroblastoma, Journal of Clinical Oncology. 2002;15;**20**(8):2142-2149

[40] Yanik GA, Villablanca J, Maris JM, et al. ^{131}I-metaiodobenzylguanidine with intensive chemotherapy and autologous stem cell transplantation for high-risk neuroblastoma. A new approaches to neuroblastoma therapy (NANT) phase II study. Biology of Blood Marrow Transplant. 2015;**21**:673-681

[41] Klingebiel T, Bader P, Bares R, et al. Treatment of neuroblastoma stage 4 with ^{131}I-meta-iodo-benzylguanidine, high dose chemotherapy and immunotherapy. A pilot study. European Journal of Cancer. 1998;**34**:1398-1402

[42] Howard JP, Maris JM, Kersun LS, et al. Tumor response and toxicity with multiple infusions of high dose ^{131}I-MIBG for refractory neuroblastoma. Pediatric Blood Cancer. 2005;**44**:232-239

[43] Matthay KK, Quach A, Huberty J, et al. Iodine-131-metaiodobenzylguanidine double infusion with autologous stem cell rescue for neuroblastoma. A new approaches to neuroblastoma therapy phase 1 study. Journal of Clinical Oncology. 2009;**27**:1020-1025

[44] Johnson K, McGlynn B, Saggio J, et al. The safety and efficacy of tandem ^{131}I-metaiodobenzylguanidine infusions in relapsed/refractory neuroblastoma. Pediatric Blood Cancer. 2011;**57**:1124-1129

[45] Wilson JS, Gaines JE, Moroz V, et al. A systematic review of ^{131}I-metaiodobenzylguanidine molecular therapy for neuroblastoma. European Journal of Cancer. 2014;**50**:801-815

[46] Mastrangelo R, Tornesello A, Lasorella A, et al. Optimal use of the 131-I-metaiodobenzylguanidine and cisplatin combination in advanced neuroblastoma. Journal of Neuro-Oncology. 1997;**31**:153-158

[47] Meco D, Lasorella A, Riccardi A, et al. Influence of cisplatin and doxorubicin on ^{125}I-metaiodobenzylguanidine uptake in human neuroblastoma cell lines. European Journal of Cancer. 1999;**35**:1227-1234

[48] Hoefnagel CA, De Kraker J, Valdes-Olmos RA, et al. ^{131}I-MIBG as a first line treatment in high-risk neuroblastoma patients. Nuclear Medicine Communications. 1994;**15**:712-717

[49] De Kraker J, Hoefnagel KA, Verschuur AC, et al. Iodine-131-metaiodobenxylguanidine as initial induction therapy in stage 4 neuroblastoma patients over 1 year of age. European Journal of Cancer. 2008;**44**:551-556

[50] Bleeker G, Schoot RA, Caron HN, et al. Toxicity of upfront ^{131}I-metaiodobenzylguanidine (^{131}I-MIBG) therapy in newly diagnosed neuroblastoma patients: A retrospective review. European Journal of Nuclear Medicine and Molecular Imaging. 2013;**40**:1711-1717

[51] Kraal KC, Tytgat GA, van Eck-Smit BL, et al. Up front treatment of high-risk neuroblastoma with a combination of ^{131}I-MIBG and topotecan. Pediatric Blood Cancer. 2015;**62**:1886-1891

[52] Weyl Ben-Arush M, Ben Barak A, Bar-Deroma R. Targeted therapy with low doses of ^{131}I-MIBG is effective for disease palliation in highly refractory neuroblastoma. Israel Medicine Association Journal. 2013;**15**:31-34

[53] De Lellis RA, Lloyd RV, Heitz PU, et al. World Health Organization classification of tumours. Pathology and Genetics of Tumours of Endocrine Organs. Lyon: IARC Press; 2004

[54] Pacak K, Keiser H, Eisenhofer G. Pheochromocytoma. In: De Groot LJ, Jameson JL, editors. Textbook of Endocrinology. Philadelphia: Elsevier Saunders Inc; 2005. pp. 2501-2534

[55] Chrisoulidou A, Kaltsas G, Ilias I, et al. The diagnosis and management of malignant phaeochromocytoma and paraganglioma. Endocrine Related Cancer. 2007;**14**:569-585

[56] Granger JK, Houn HY. Head and neck paragangliomas: A clinicopathologic study with DNA flow cytometric analysis. Southern Medical Journal. 1990;**83**:1407-1412

[57] Linnoila RI, Keiser HR, Steinberg SM, et al. Histopathology of benign versus malignant sympathoadrenal paragangliomas: Clinicopathologic study of 120 cases including unusual histologic features. Human Pathology. 1990;**21**:1168-1180

[58] Scholz T, Schulz C, Klose S, et al. Diagnostic management of benign and malignant pheochromocytoma. Experimental and Clinical Endocrinology & Diabetes. 2007;**115**: 155-159

[59] Fitzgerald PA, Goldsby RE, Huberty JP, et al. Malignant pheochromocytomas and paragangliomas: A phase II study of therapy with high-dose ^{131}I-metaiodobenzylguanidine (^{131}IMIBG). Annals of the New York Academy of Sciences. 2006;**1073**:465-490

[60] Sisson JC, Shapiro B, Beierwaltes WH, et al. Radiopharmaceutical treatment of malignant pheochromocytoma. Journal of Nuclear Medicine. 1984;**25**:197-206

[61] Taggart D, Dubois S, Matthay KK. Radiolabeled metaiodobenzylguanidine for imaging and therapy of neuroblastoma. Quarterly Journal of Nuclear Medicine and Molecular Imaging. 2008;**52**(4):403-418

[62] Loh KC, Fitzgerald PA, Matthay KK, et al. The treatment of malignant metaiodobenzylguanidine (I-131-MIBG): A comprehensive review of 116 reported patients. Journal of Endocrinology Investigation. 1997;**20**(11):648-658

[63] Safford SD, Coleman E, Gockerman JP, et al. Iodine-131 metaiodobenzylguanidine is an effective treatment for malignant pheochromocytoma and paraganglioma. Surgery. 2003;**134**:956-962

[64] van Hulsteijn LT, Niemeijer ND, Dekkers OM, Corssmit EP. (131)I-MIBG therapy for malignant paraganglioma and phaeochromocytoma: Systematic review and meta-analysis. Clinical Endocrinology (Oxford). 2014;**80**:487-501

[65] Hoefnagel CA, Voûte PA, de Kraker J, Marcuse HR, Radionuclide diagnosis and therapy of neural crest tumors using iodine-131 metaiodobenzylguanidine. Journal of Nuclear Medicine. 1987;**28**:308-314

[66] Clarke SE, Lazarus CR, Edwards S. Scintigraphy and treatment of medullary carcinoma of the thyroid with iodine-131 metaiodobenzylguanidine. Journal of Nuclear Medicine. 1987;**28**:1820-1825

[67] Kratochwil C, Giesel FL. Radionuclide therapy of endocrine-related cancer. Radiologe. 2014;**54**:1007-1015

[68] Safford SD, Coleman RE, Gockerman JP, et al. Iodine-131 metaiodobenzylguanidine treatment for metastatic carcinoid. Results in 98 patients. Cancer. 2004;**101**:1987-1993

[69] Mukherjee JJ, Kaltsas GA, Islam N, et al. Treatment of metastatic carcinoid tumours, phaeochromocytoma, paraganglioma and medullary carcinoma of the thyroid with I-131-meta-iodobenzylguanidine (I-131-MIBG). Clinical Endocrinology. 2001;**55**:47-60

[70] Gedik GK, Hoefnagel CA, Bais E, et al. ^{131}I-MIBG therapy in metastatic phaeochromocytoma and paraganglioma. European Journal of Nuclear Medicine and Molecular Imaging. 2008;**35**:725-733

[71] Whittle SB, Smith V, Doherty E, Zhao S, McCarty S, Zage PE. Overview and recent advances in the treatment of neuroblastoma. Expert Review of Anticancer Therapy. 2017. DOİ: 10.1080/14737140.2017.1285230. 2017 ;**17**:369-386

[72] Rose B, Matthay KK, Price D, et al. High-dose I-131-metaiodobenzylguanidine therapy for 12 patients with malignant pheochromocytoma. Cancer. 2003;**98**:239-248

[73] Rutherford MA, Rankin AJ, Yates TM, et al. Management of metastatic phaeochromocytoma and paraganglioma: Use of iodine-131-meta-iodobenzylguanidine therapy in a tertiary referral centre. QJM. 2015;**108**:361-368

[74] Modak S, Pandit-Taskar N, Kushner BH, et al. Transient sialadenitis: A complication of ^{131}I-metaiodobenzylguanidine therapy. Pediatric Blood Cancer. 2008;**50**:1271-1273

[75] DuBois SG, Messina J, Maris JM, Huberty J, Glidden DV, Veatch J, Charron M, Hawkins R, Matthay KK. Hematologic toxicity of high-dose iodine-131-metaiodobenzylguanidine therapy for advanced neuroblastoma. Journal of Clinical Oncology. 2004;**22**:2452-2460

[76] Shusterman S, Grant FD, Lorenzen W, et al. Iodine-131-labeled Meta-iodobenzylguanidine therapy of children with neuroblastoma: Program planning and initial experience. Seminars in Nuclear Medicine. 2011;**41**:354-363

[77] Picco P, Garaventa A, Claudiani F, et al. Primary hypothyroidism as a consequence of 131-I-metaiodobenzylguanidine treatment for children with neuroblastoma. Cancer. 1995;**76**:1662-1664

[78] Van Santen HM, De Kraker J, van Eck BL, et al. High incidence of thyroid dysfunction despite prophylaxis with potassium iodide during ^{131}I-metaiodobenzylguanidine treatment in children with neuroblastoma. Cancer. 2002;**94**:2081-2089

[79] Van Santen HM, De Kraker J, van Eck BL, et al. Improved radiation protection of the thyroid gland with thyroxine, methimazole, and potassium iodide during diagnostic and therapeutic use of radiolabeled metaiodobenzylguandine in children with neuroblastoma. Cancer. 2003;**98**:389-396

[80] Van Santen HM, De Kraker J, Vulsma T. Endocrine late effects from multimodality treatment of neuroblastoma. European Journal of Cancer. 2005;**41**:1767-1774

[81] Quach A, Ji L, Mishra V, et al. Thyroid and hepatic function after high-dose ^{131}I-metaiodobenzylguanidine (^{131}I-MIBG) therapy for neuroblastoma. Pediatric Blood Cancer. 2011;**56**:191-201

[82] Polishuck AL, DuBois SG, Hass-Kogan D, et al. Response, survival, and toxicity after iodine-131-metaiodobenzylguanidine therapy for neuroblastoma in preadolescents, adolescents, and adults. Cancer. 2011;**117**:4286-4293

[83] Garaventa A, Gambini C, Villavecchia G, et al. Second malignancies in children with neuroblastoma after combined treatment with ^{131}I-metaiodobenzylguanidine. Cancer. 2003;**97**:1332-1338

[84] Weiss B, Vora A, Huberty J, et al. Secondary myelodysplastic syndrome and leukemia following ^{131}I-metaiodobenzylguanidine therapy for relapsed neuroblastoma. Journal of Pediatric Hematology/Oncology. 2003;**25**:543-547

[85] Tonakie A, Shulkin BL, Sisson JC, et al. Radiation-induced osteosarcoma and papillary thyroid carcinoma of the thyroid. Clinical Nuclear Medicine. 2006;**31**:5-8

[86] Matthay KK, Tan JC, Villablanca JG, et al. Phase 1 dose escalation of iodine-131-metaiodobenzylguanidine with myeloablative chemotherapy and autologous stem-cell transplantation in refractory neuroblastoma: A new approaches to neuroblastoma therapy consortium study. Journal of Clinical Oncology. 2006;**24**:500-506

[87] George SL, Falzone N, Chittenden S, Kirk SJ, Lancaster D, Vaidya SJ, Mandeville H, Saran F, Pearson AD, Du Y, Meller ST, Denis-Bacelar AM, Flux GD. Individualized ^{131}I-mIBG therapy in the management of refractory and relapsed neuroblastoma. Nuclear Medicine Communication. 2016;**37**:466-472

[88] Mangner JT, Wu J-L, Wieland DM. Solid-phase exchange radioiodination of aryl iodides: Facilitation by ammonium sulfate. The Journal of Organic Chemistry. 1982;**47**:1484-1488

[89] Vaidyanathan G, Zalutsky MR. No-carrier-added synthesis of meta-[^{131}I]iodobenzylguanidine. Applied Radiation and Isotopes. 1999;**44**:621-628

[90] Hunter DH, Zhu X. Polymer-supported radiopharmaceuticals: [^{131}I] MIBG and [^{123}I] MIBG. Journal of Labelled Compounds and Radiopharmaceuticals. 1999;**42**:653-661

[91] James O, Coleman RE: Radioiodinated MIBG in paraganglioma and pheochromocytoma: Previous results and early experiences using nocarrier-added MIBG. Nuclear Medicine and Biology. 2009;**35**:63-76

Chapter 4

Radionuclide Pain Palliation Treatment and Radiosynovectomy

Elgin Özkan

Additional information is available at the end of the chapter

http://dx.doi.org/10.5772/intechopen.68623

Abstract

The main nuclear medicine palliation treatment methods are radionuclide pain palliation treatment in cases of disseminated painful bone metastases and radiosynovectomy in inflammatory arthritis cases. Both methods can be easily administered and do not require long-term hospitalization. They are reliable with high palliation value and low complication rates.

Keywords: radiosynovectomy, radionuclide pain palliation treatment, therapy response

1. Radionuclide pain palliation treatment

1.1. Introduction

Painful bone metastases are one of the most common causes of morbidity in metastatic cancer patients. The vast majority of these patients need multiple medical treatments. The most common tumors, which cause painful bone metastases, are breast, prostate, lung, and renal tumors [1]. If not diagnosed or sufficiently treated, painful bone metastases cause severe pain, spinal cord compression, hypercalcemia, and pathological fractures. In many studies, a direct correlation has been determined between bone metastasis load and survival [2]. The majority of bone metastases are localized in the axial skeleton due to the presence of bone marrow [3]. Generally, bone metastases are classified as osteoblastic, osteolytic, or mixed type. Although some tumors have pure blastic or lytic metastases, the metastases of many tumors are of mixed phenotype [4].

Pain associated with bone metastases is generally seen in two different forms. The nature of the first is related with bone remodeling, and chronic pain due to inflammatory reaction in and around the metastatic focus. The nature of the second type of pain is more severe and is acute pain exacerbated by physical activity or patient position [5, 6]. Non-steroid or narcotic analgesics and external beam radiotherapy (EBRT) are the most commonly used therapy methods for the palliation of metastatic bone pain [7]. Although conventional radiotherapy is an effective method in the palliation of symptoms from bone metastasis, many patients have painful bone metastases in many different regions of the skeletal system [8]. Although wide-field radiations such as hemibody radiotherapy are also effective, they are not preferred due to technical difficulties and radiation toxicity [9, 10]. Systemic therapy management should be preferred for patients with diffuse symptomatic bone involvement. In these patients, intravenous bisphosphonates may have a role in the reduction of the development of complications.

1.2. Treatment

In the last few decades, different radionuclides have been used for radionuclide pain palliation. Radionuclides are usually administered intravenously and are quickly localized in regions of active bone reaction and remodeling. Radionuclide pain palliation treatment is indicated in patients with multiple bone metastases shown on bone scintigraphy and in cases that cannot be treated with non-steroidal or narcotic analgesics or who are resistant to these treatments [11]. In the presence of epidural spinal cord pressure, active pathological fracture, renal failure, pregnancy, and lactation, treatment is not recommended. Patients with uncontrolled non-skeletal metastasis, asymptomatic bone metastases, ≤3 bone metastases, purely osteolytic lesions, and patients with a shorter life expectancy (<2 months) are relatively contraindicated. The physical properties of radionuclides used in radionuclide pain palliation are shown in **Table 1**.

Radionuclide	Half life (days)	Decay type	Mean energy (keV)	Mean penetration depth (mm)	Gamma ray
Phosphor-32 [P-32]	14.3	β-	695	3.0	Yok
Strontium-89 [Sr-89]	50.5	β-	580	2.4	Yok
Samarium-153 [Sm-153]	1.9	β-	233	0.5	Var
Renium-186 [Re-186]	3.7	β-	349	1.1	Var
Renium-188 [Re-188]	0.7	β-	2120	3.0	Var
Tin-177m [Sn-177m]	13.6	CE	127	<0.1	Yok
Radium-223 [Ra-223]	11.4	α	5850	<0.1	Var

β- = beta ray, CE = conversion electron, α = alpha ray.

Table 1. The physical properties of the radionuclides used in pain palliation treatment.

The radionuclides used in radionuclide pain palliation act through two main mechanisms. The first group is attracted to calcium and directly localizes to the bone matrix. The other group is applied as chelate with organic phosphates and is added to the bone matrix [11]. Gama-emitting radionuclides provide post-therapy imaging on gamma cameras.

1.3. Follow-up

No special radiation safety precaution is necessary because the emission rates of the radionuclides used for pain palliation are very low. Therefore, hospitalization is not required for treatment. The patient can be quickly mobilized after several hours of treatment. The administration takes approximately 1 min as an intravenous injection followed by a 20–30-ml saline wash through the vein. The patient is then advised to take oral hydration and make frequent toilet trips for a few hours. Following the treatment, a weekly complete blood count for an 8-week period is recommended. Transient myelosuppression can be monitored. Thrombocytopenia is the most common finding, which is characterized by a 40–60% decrease in platelet count compared to the baseline value. Most cases have grade 1 or 2 toxicity. Neutropenia and anemia are rare.

A decrease in the pain of the patient is expected at 1–3 weeks after treatment, although it varies according to the radionuclide used [12]. Positive response to therapy has been reported as 60–92%, although it can vary according to the primary malignancy and the spread of the disease [13–21]. Flare phenomena can be observed as an increase in pain which is severe but usually self-limiting during 24–48 h after treatment. Patients with flare phenomena have been shown to have a better response rate to treatment compared to those where it is not experienced. Palliation times of up to 6 months have been reported following radionuclide treatment. Different pain-scoring systems and patient questionnaires can be used to evaluate treatment response [22]. It is also helpful to evaluate the patient's narcotic analgesic needs. Pain scoring systems and quality of life questionnaires that can be used for this purpose are presented in **Table 2**.

Serafini et al. compared Sm-153 EDTMP with a placebo in bone metastases of solid tumor in a randomized, prospective study and showed that patients receiving higher doses of Sm-153 responded better at all times (1–4 weeks) than those who had received the placebo. In two-thirds of the patients evaluated, the response to treatment was in the fourth week and palliation continued until the 16th week [23].

Visual Analog Scale for Pain (VAS Pain)
Numeric Rating Scale for Pain (NRS Pain)
McGill Pain Questionnaire (MPQ)
Short-form McGill Pain Questionnaire (SF-MPQ)
Chronic Pain Grade Scale (CPGS)
Short Form-36 Bodily Pain Scale (SF-36 BPS)
Physician's Global Assessment of Pain (PGA)

Table 2. The scoring systems that can be used in the evaluation of pain palliation pretreatment and of the response to treatment.

Sartor et al. reported a significantly better objective response rate in a double-blind randomized study of patients with bone metastasis of prostate cancer where Sm-153 was compared with a placebo. The objective response rates of the Sm-153 group were reported to be better [24]. Several studies have reported that the use of Sm-153 in repeated doses and in combination with different chemotherapy regimes was more reliable [25–28]. During treatment with Sr-89 in prostate cancer cases, a single-dose relationship was shown and doses reaching 10.8 mCi were not determined to affect survival [29]. However, application combined with chemotherapy was determined to remove both the efficacy of pain palliation and survival [30–32]. In two randomized studies, Sr-89 and EBRT were applied alone and similar rates of pain palliation were obtained, but it was shown that after treatment with Sr-89, there was a lower possibility of the development of new painful bone metastasis [33, 34]. Radium-223 has started to be used in recent years, and according to the results of the first studies, it is a radionuclide that extends survival in addition to providing pain palliation. In prostate cancer cases, it has been shown to provide prolonged survival, and reduced levels of PSA and ALP compared to a placebo and no difference has been observed in hematological toxicity [35].

In summary, radionuclide pain palliation treatment is an effective method in patients with osteoblastic, widespread painful bone metastasis. The simple and systemic application provides the significant advantage of allowing treatment of all the painful lesions of the patient. It is a safe method with low rates of side effects even when applied at repeated doses or combined with different chemotherapy regimes.

2. Radiosynovectomy

2.1. Introduction

The use of radionuclides was first described in 1963 with the use of Au-198 in the treatment of persistent knee effusion in arthritis treatment. However, as Au-198 particles are very small, their leakage outside the knee joint caused severe clinical side effects [36]. In subsequent years, Yttrium-90 [Y-90], colloidal P-32, and Re-186 sulfide colloid were radionuclides which came to be often used for radiosynovectomy. In the last 20 years, Erbium-169 citrate [Er-169] has started to be used in small joints [37–39].

Due to proliferation and hyperperfusion in synovial tissue in inflammatory arthritis, there is effusion, macrophage accumulation, and the expression of inflammatory cytokines in the joint space. Consequently, pain, loss of movement, and in long term, arthrosis are observed in the affected joint. Radiosynovectomy is effective in approximately 80% of rheumatoid arthritis patients. In developed countries, there is increasing use of radiosynovectomy because of pain and restricted movement in osteoarthritic joints which occur with increasing life expectancies. The current most common indications for application are rheumatoid arthritis, psoriatic arthritis, osteoarthritis, hemophilic arthritis, and villonodular synovitis. The radionuclides widely used for radiosynovectomy and their physical properties are shown in **Table 3**. Due to the energy and soft-tissue penetration properties, Er-169 is used in small joints, Re-186 and P-32 in medium-sized joints, and Y-90 in large joints [40, 41].

Radionuclide	Half life (days)	Soft-tissue penetration (mm)	Energy (MeV)
Er-169	9.5	0.3–1	0.34
Re-186	13.7	1.2–3.7	0.98
Au-198	2.7	1.2–3.6	0.96β–0.41γ

Table 3. The physical properties of the radionuclides used for radiosynovectomy.

2.2. Treatment

In radiosynovectomy, particles of 0.05–2 μm in size are applied directly into the joint space. After application, the particles reaching the synovia are phagocytized by macrophages and other inflammatory cells. The absorption by the synovia of a dose of approximately 100-Gy radiation results in synovectomy similar to surgical synovectomy. As beta particles have tissue penetration up to a maximum of 10 mm, the surrounding soft tissues are protected from radiation damage [42]. Pregnancy, breastfeeding, local infection, massive hemarthrosis, or ruptured Baker cyst are contraindications for radiosynovectomy.

2.3. Follow-up

After treatment, it is recommended that the joint is immobilized for 48 h. If a sufficient response is not observed after the first application, radiosynovectomy can be reapplied three times at a 3-month interval. Repeated doses are more effective than a single, high-dose application. Side effects following radiosynovectomy have been reported to be extremely rarely. These may include infection, thrombosis, and skin necrosis caused by extra-articular application [43]. To prevent thrombosis, the use of heparin is recommended in the immobilization period. The response to treatment is closely related to the degree of synovitis, the level of arthrosis pre-treatment, and in rheumatoid arthritis cases, the level of systemic inflammation. The highest response rates have been reported in cases of hemophilic arthritis [44, 45]. If treatment is applied in the early stages of arthrosis, the success rates are high, with response rates of 73% reported in cases of early stage rheumatoid arthritis [46]. In cases of radiosynovectomy applied to the knee joint because of osteoarthritis, the response rate has been reported as 40–85% [46].

These serious differences in rates in the evaluation of treatment response are due to the fact that objective scoring systems have not been used. In the evaluation of the response to treatment following radiosynovectomy, physical examination, clinical scoring systems, and radiological response criteria can be used. In the physical examination, swelling in the joint, pain, restricted movement, and weakness are evaluated as the response to treatment. In the clinical scoring system, treatment response is classified as excellent, good, fair, and ineffective. In a report of this scoring system applied to 577 patients, excellent and good responses were obtained in the knee joint in 57%, in the shoulder joint in 63%, the elbow in 61%, the wrist in 64%, finger joints in 54%, and metacarpophalangeal joints in 54% [47].

Another parameter used in the evaluation of response following radiosynovectomy is the Visual Analog Scale for Pain (VAS Pain). The VAS score of rheumatoid arthritis patients at 6 months after radiosynovectomy has been determined to be improved by three stages compared to the pretreatment score [48]. As a more objective evaluation of response following radiosynovectomy, blood pool phase activity involvement on three-phase Tc-99m MDP bone scintigraphy can be used. Response has been determined in small joints at 81% and in large joints at 69% with Tc-99m MDP bone scintigraphy following radiosynovectomy [49]. Unlike cases of pigmented villonodular synovitis, the application of radiosynovectomy after surgical synovectomy has been shown to be more effective in resistant cases [50].

In conclusion, when the radionuclide is selected appropriate to the size of the joint, radiosynovectomy is a safe option in the treatment of inflammatory arthritis with high success and low complication rates.

Author details

Elgin Özkan

Address all correspondence to: ozkanelgin@yahoo.com

Ankara University Medical School, Department of Nuclear Medicine, Ankara, Turkey

References

[1] Paes FM, Serafini AN. Systemic metabolic radiopharmaceutical therapy in the treatment of metastatic bone pain. Seminars in Nuclear Medicine. 2010;40:89-104

[2] Soloway MS, Hardeman SW, Hickey D, et al. Stratification of patients with metastatic prostate cancer based on extent of disease on initial bone scan. Cancer. 1988;61:195-202

[3] Cleeland CS. Cancer-related symptoms. Seminars in Radiation Oncology. 2000;10:175-190

[4] Stoll BA. Natural history, prognosis, and staging of bone metastases. In: Szoll BA, Parboo S, editors. Bone Metastases: Monitoring and Treatment. New York, NY: Raven; 1983. pp. 1-20

[5] Horvat AG, Kovač V, Strojan P. Radiotherapy in palliative treatment of painful bone metastases. Radiological Oncology. 2009;43:213-224

[6] Portenoy RK, Payne D, Jacobsen P. Breakthrough pain: Characteristics and impact in patients with cancer pain. Pain. 1999;81:129-134

[7] Lutz S, Berk L, Chang E, et al. Palliative radiotherapy for bone metastases: An ASTRO evidence-based guideline. International Journal of Radiation Oncology, Biology, Physics. 2011;79:965-976

[8] Tong D, Gillick L, Hendrickson FR. The palliation of symptomatic osseous metastases: Final results of the Study by the Radiation Therapy Oncology Group. Cancer. 1982;50:893-899

[9] Poulter CA, Cosmatos D, Rubin P, et al. A report of RTOG 8206: A phase III study of whether the addition of single dose hemibody irradiation to standard fractionated local field irradiation is more effective than local field irradiation alone in the treatment of symptomatic osseous metastases. International Journal of Radiation Oncology, Biology, Physics. 1992;23:207-214

[10] Kuban DA, Delbridge T, el-Mahdi AM, et al. Half-body irradiation for treatment of widely metastatic adenocarcinoma of the prostate. Journal of Urology.1989;141:572-574

[11] Michael Tomblyn, MD, MS. The role of bone-seeking radionuclides in the palliative treatment of patients with painful osteoblastic skeletal metastases. Cancer Control. 2012;19:137-144

[12] Collins C, Eary JF, Donaldson G, et al. Samarium-153-EDTMP in bone metastases of hormone refractory prostate carcinoma: A phase I/II trial. Journal of Nuclear Medicine. 1993;34:1839-1844

[13] Dolezal J. Systemic radionuclide therapy with samarium-153-EDTMP for painful bone metastases. Nuclear Medicine Review Central & Eastern Europe. 2000;3:161-163

[14] Dolezal J, Vizda J, Odrazka K. Prospective evaluation of samarium-153-EDTMP radionuclide treatment for bone metastases in patients with hormone-refractory prostate cancer. Urologia Internationalis. 2007;78:50-57

[15] Tian JH, Zhang JM, Hou QT, et al. Multicentre trial on the efficacy and toxicity of single-dose samarium-153-ethylene diamine tetramethylene phosphonate as a palliative treatment for painful skeletal metastases in China. European Journal of Nuclear Medicine. 1999;26:2-7

[16] Etchebehere EC, Pereira Neto CA, Lima MC, et al. Treatment of bone pain secondary to metastases using samarium-153-EDTMP. Sao Paulo Medical Journal. 2004;122:208-212

[17] Sapienza MT, Ono CR, Guimarães MI, et al. Retrospective evaluation of bone pain palliation after samarium-153-EDTMP therapy. Revisto do Hospital das Clinicas Faculdade de Medicina Sao Paulo. 2004;59:321-328

[18] Fuster D, Herranz D, Vidal-Sicart S, et al. Usefulness of strontium-89 for bone pain palliation in metastatic breast cancer patients. Nuclear Medicine Communications. 2000;21: 623-626

[19] Kraeber-Bodéré F, Campion L, Rousseau C, et al. Treatment of bone metastases of prostate cancer with strontium-89 chloride: Efficacy in relation to the degree of bone involvement. European Journal of Nuclear Medicine. 2000;27:1487-1493

[20] Ashayeri E, Omogbehin A, Sridhar R, et al. Strontium 89 in the treatment of pain due to diffuse osseous metastases: A university hospital experience. Journal of the National Medical Association. 2002;94:706-711

[21] Gunawardana DH, Lichtenstein M, Better N, et al. Results of strontium-89 therapy in patients with prostate cancer resistant to chemotherapy. Clinical Nuclear Medicine. 2004;29:81-85

[22] Liepe K, Kotzerke J. A comparative study of 188Re-HEDP, 186Re-HEDP, 153Sm-EDTMP and 89Sr in the treatment of painful skeletal metastases. Nuclear Medicine Communications. 2007;28:623-630

[23] Serafini AN, Houston SJ, Resche I, et al. Palliation of pain associated with metastatic bone cancer using samarium-153 lexidronam: A double-blind placebo-controlled clinical trial. Journal of Clinical Oncology. 1998;16:1574-1581

[24] Sartor O, Reid RH, Hoskin PJ, et al. Samarium-153-lexidronam complex for treatment of painful bone metastases in hormone-refractory prostate cancer. Urology. 2004;63:940-945

[25] Menda Y, Bushnell DL, Williams RD, et al. Efficacy and safety of repeated samarium-153 lexidronam treatment in a patient with prostate cancer and metastatic bone pain. Clinical Nuclear Medicine. 2000;25:698-700

[26] Morris MJ, Pandit-Taskar N, Carrasquillo J, et al. Phase I study of samarium-153 lexidronam with docetaxel in castration-resistant metastatic prostate cancer. Journal of Clinical Oncology. 2009;27:2436-2442

[27] Tu SM, Mathew P, Wong FC, et al. Phase I study of concurrent weekly docetaxel and repeated samarium-153 lexidronam in patients with castration-resistant metastatic prostate cancer. Journal of Clinical Oncology. 2009;27:3319-3324

[28] Fizazi K, Beuzeboc P, Lumbroso J, et al. Phase II trial of consolidation docetaxel and samarium-153 in patients with bone metastases from castration-resistant prostate cancer. Journal of Clinical Oncology. 2009;27:2429-2435

[29] Porter AT, McEwan AJ, Powe JE, et al. Results of a randomized phase III trial to evaluate the efficacy of strontium-89 adjuvant to local field external beam irradiation in the management of endocrine resistant metastatic prostate cancer. International Journal of Radiation Oncology, Biology, Physics. 1993;25:805-813

[30] Sciuto R, Maini CL, Tofani A, et al. Radiosensitization with lowdose carboplatin enhances pain palliation in radioisotope therapy with strontium-89. Nuclear Medicine Communication. 1996;17:799-804

[31] Sciuto R, Festa A, Rea S, et al. Effects of low-dose cisplatin on 89Sr therapy for painful bone metastases from prostate cancer: A randomized clinical trial. Journal of Nuclear Medicine. 2002;43:79-86

[32] Tu SM, Millikan RE, Mengistu B, et al. Bone-targeted therapy for advanced androgen-independent carcinoma of the prostate: A randomised phase II trial. Lancet. 2001;357:336-341

[33] Oosterhof GO, Roberts JT, de Reijke TM, et al. Strontium [89] chloride versus palliative local field radiotherapy in patients with hormonal escaped prostate cancer: A phase III study of the European Organisation for Research and Treatment of Cancer, Genitourinary Group. European Urology. 2003;44:519-526

[34] Quilty PM, Kirk D, Bolger JJ, et al. A comparison of the palliative effects of strontium-89 and external beam radiotherapy in metastatic prostate cancer. Radiotherapy Oncology. 1994;31:33-40

[35] Nilsson S, Franzén L, Parker C, et al. Bone-targeted radium-223 in symptomatic, hormone-refractory prostate cancer: A randomised, multicentre, placebo-controlled phase II study. Lancet Oncology. 2007;8(7):587-594

[36] Knut L. Radiosynovectomy in the therapeutic management of arthritis. World Journal of Nuclear Medicine. 2015 Jan–Apr;14(1):10-15

[37] Ansell BM, Crook A, Mallard JR, Bywaters EG. Evaluation of intra-articular colloidal gold au 198 in the treatment of persistent knee effusions. Annals of the Rheumatic Diseases. 1963;22:435-439

[38] Kerschbaumer F, Bauer R, Falser N, Altmann H. Effects and side effects of radiosynovectomy with Yttrium 90 on rheumatic joint cartilage. Archives of Orthopaedic and Trauma Surgery. 1979;93:95-102

[39] Howson MP, Shepard NL, Mitchell NS. Colloidal chromic phosphate ^{32}P synovectomy in antigen-induced arthritis in the rabbit. Clinical Orthopaedics and Related Research. 1988;229:283-293

[40] Soroa VE, del Huerto Velázquez Espeche M, Giannone C, Caviglia H, Galatros G, Fernández D, et al. Effects of radiosynovectomy with p-32 colloid therapy in hemophilia and rheumatoid arthritis. Cancer Biotherapy and Radiopharmaceuticals. 2005;20:344-348

[41] Liepe K. Efficacy of radiosynovectomy in rheumatoid arthritis. Rheumatology International. 2012;32:3219-3224

[42] Bowring CS, Keeling DH. Absorbed radiation dose in radiation synovectomy. British Journal of Radiology. 1978;51:836-837

[43] Kampen WU, Matis E, Czech N, Soti Z, Gratz S, Henze E. Serious complications after radiosynoviorthesis. Survey on frequency and treatment modalities. Nuklearmedizin. 2006;45:262-268

[44] Kresnik E, Mikosch P, Gallowitsch HJ, Jesenko R, Just H, Kogler D, et al. Clinical outcome of radiosynoviorthesis: A meta-analysis including 2190 treated joints. Nuclear Medicine Communications. 2002;23:683-688

[45] Siegel HJ, Luck JV, Jr, Siegel ME, Quinones C. Phosphate-32 colloid radiosynovectomy in hemophilia: Outcome of 125 procedures. Clinical Orthopeadics and Related Research. 2001;392:409-417

[46] Mathew P, Talbut DC, Frogameni A, Singer D, Chrissos M, Khuder S, et al. Isotopic synovectomy with P-32 in paediatric patients with haemophilia. Haemophilia. 2000;6:547-555

[47] Deutsch E, Brodack JW, Deutsch KF. Radiation synovectomy revisited. European Journal of Nuclear Medicine. 1993;20:1113-1127

[48] Zagnun J, Liepe K, Soroa VE, Barrenechea E, Gaudiano J, Solav SV, et al. Management of haemarthrosis applying radiosynovectomy in haemophilia patients with emphasis on developing countries. European Journal of Nuclear Medicine. 2007;34:439

[49] Zuderman L, Liepe K, Zöphel K, Andreeff M, Kotzerke J, Luboldt W. Radiosynoviorthesis [RSO]: Influencing factors and therapy monitoring. Annals in Nuclear Medicine. 2008;22:735-741

[50] Oztemür Z, Bulut O, Korkmaz M, Gölge UH, Oztürk H, Tezeren G, et al. Surgical synovectomy combined with yttrium 90 in patients with recurrent joint synovitis. Rheumatology International. 2013;33:1321-1326

Chapter 5

Yttrium-90 Selective Internal Radiation Therapy for Liver Tumors

Umut Elboga

Additional information is available at the end of the chapter

http://dx.doi.org/10.5772/intechopen.69328

Abstract

The aim of this chapter to evaluate the effects of yttrium-90 (Y-90) radioembolization on primary and metastatic liver tumors with delivering implantable radioactive microspheres into branches of hepatic arteries that feed liver tumors to provide a high dose of targeted radiation to tumor tissue. Yttrium-90 (Y-90), a high-energetic beta emitter, is the most preferred radionuclide, which is used to label microspheres. The principle of this therapeutic option depends on the different blood sources of healthy and malign cells in liver. In liver primary or metastatic tumor cells, most of the blood is supplied via the hepatic artery. Arterial supply of malignant liver tumors in contrast with mostly portal venous supply of normal hepatocytes as well as excess amount of arterial neovascularization in the tumor bed. Therefore, intra-arterial radionuclide therapy can provide very high radiation exposure to tumor tissue, which is impossible to reach with external radiation therapy due to serious side effects. Y-90 microsphere therapy is an efficient and safe locoregional therapeutic option for unresectable primary and metastatic liver tumors.

Keywords: yttrium-90, internal radiation therapy, liver tumor

1. Introduction

Yttrium-90 (Y-90) microsphere therapy of liver tumors is an internal radiotherapy method by administering Y-90 radiopharmaceutical loaded microspheres that emit therapeutic beta-radiation from the relevant branch feeding the hepatic arterial tumor through femoral artery. The theoretical basis of treatment based on the fact of the different blood sources of healthy and malign cells in liver.

Most of the blood of healthy hepatocytes is supplied from the portal venous system, but a very small part is fed from the hepatic artery. In liver primary or metastatic tumor cells, most of the blood is supplied via the hepatic artery. Based on this different nutritional pathway between benign and malignant cells in the liver, when microspheres that contain high dose radiation applied from hepatic artery intra-arterially, a very large portion of the applied radiation is targeted directly to the tumor cells; and healthy cells are protected as long as they are protected from radiation damage.

Since the intra-arterial delivery route is a local application, the radiomicrospheres cannot reach the extrahepatic tissues if there is no vessel shunt and as a result of this side effects based on treatments are seen very rare compared to other oncologic treatments [1, 2].

Y-90 used as a radiation source for intra-arterial Y-90 microsphere treatment is a pure beta-emitter radionuclide with a physical half-life of 64.2 hours. Tissue permeability of Y-90 microspheres is very low (mean 2.5 mm and maximum 10 mm), and therefore, if targeted correctly, is unlikely to cause harmful side effects to the surrounding tissues. The mean beta-particle energy given to tumor cells in Y-90 microsphere treatment is quite high and is around 2.28 MeV. Accordingly, high dose radiation therapy is provided in targeted tumor cells [1–4].

Two types of radiomicrospheres are used in the treatment of intra-arterial Y90-microspheres: resin-based (Y90-resin microspheres SIRSphere®, Sirtex Medical Europe, Bonn, Germany) and glass-based (Y90-glass microspheres Therasphere®, MDS Nordion, Toronto, Canada). Despite having similar biological behaviors, the physical properties of resin and glass radiomicrospheres are different, and the methods of treatment selection and application differ accordingly [3, 4] (**Table 1**).

	Resin radiomicrosphere	Glass radiomicrosphere
Diameter	22 ± 10 μm	32 ± 10 μm
Density	1.6 g/dL	3.6 g/dL
Average microsphere number (for the same treatment dose)	60 million/3 GBq	1.2 million/3 GBq
Average activity amount per microsphere	50 GBq	2500 GBq

Table 1. Some physical properties of commercial microspheres used in intra-arterial Y-90 microsphere treatment.

2. Patient evaluation

Intra-arterial Y-90 microspheres in liver tumors are an effective and safe treatment modality for primary and metastatic tumors that cannot be treated surgically, but each patient is not eligible for this treatment. For the efficiency and safety of the treatment, it is necessary to apply the patient selection steps very carefully. The evaluation and application of Y-90 microsphere therapy require a multidisciplinary approach. As a discipline applying nuclear medicine and interventional radiology to this approach, the relevant clinical branch patients, especially medical oncology, gastroenterology, and general surgery, should take an active role in evaluating the patient's treatment adequacy as the disciplines that direct this treatment.

Pretreatment assessment is mainly carried out in two stages. During the initial evaluation stage, the patient's general condition, physical examination, laboratory, and imaging findings are examined in detail. Hepatic angiography and hepatic artery perfusion scintigraphy are used for second-stage evaluation.

In order to receive intra-arterial Y-90 microspheres, the liver functional reserve must be such that the patient's life can be survived after treatment. In this context, the first preferred biochemical criteria for evaluating the suitability of treatment is being the normal upper limits of total bilirubin <2 g/L, albumin >3 g/dL, Alanine Aminotransferase (ALT) and Aspartate Aminotransferase (AST) 5 times lower. In addition to this for some assessments such as invasion level of tumor to the liver, vascularization of tumor, whether vascular structures invaded by tumor or not, neighborhood of tumor to main vascular structures and large bile ducts computerized tomography (CT) or magnetic resonance imaging (MRI) are examined in detail.

If appropriate indications are available for assessment of disease prevalence and phase, F-18 fluorodeoxyglucose positron emission tomography (FDG PET/CT) imaging is used for whole body. In general, in patients with widespread extrahepatic disease and in those patients whose life expectancy is less than 3 months, treatment is not preferred except in very special cases.

In addition to these assessments, the interventional radiology department evaluates the advantages and disadvantages of Y-90 microsphere treatment according to whether alternative vascular access is possible or not in the first stage and other alternative interventional treatments. Clinical disciplines that refer the patient to this treatment should also consider in detail whether there is a surgical chance of the patient's tumor in the first stage and evaluation of treatment prioritization in patients who require systemic treatment in addition to the local treatment approach [1, 4].

In the pretreatment evaluation, if it is decided as a result of the above-mentioned multidisciplinary studies, the evaluation is passed to the second stage. This stage includes hepatic angiography in the interventional radiology department and intra-arterial hepatic artery perfusion scintigraphy performed on the same day in the nuclear medicine department. This stage includes hepatic angiography in the interventional radiology department and intra-arterial hepatic artery perfusion scintigraphy performed on the same day in the nuclear medicine department.

Hepatic angiography: Arterial vascularization of the liver occurs directly comes from the celiac truncus in 55–65% of cases. Mostly celiac truncus are divided into three branches such as splenic artery, left gastric artery, and arteria hepatis communis. Up to 90% of cases, gastroduodenal artery arises from the arteria hepatis communis and after this branching it is named as arteria hepatica propria. Depending on some developmental anomalies that may occur in the embryonic period, arterial vascularization of the entire liver or related segment of the liver may be obtained from a different source except the arterial hepatis propria in some cases and this is called "replaced hepatic artery," At the same time, even though a portion of the liver may be fed from the same lob or from arteria hepatis propria it may also be fed from an aberrant artery and this artery called as "accessory artery."

If the radiomicrospheres are directed to the lobe where the tumor is or selectively to the segment in the liver, there is a high likelihood of escape to the gastrointestinal tract due to feeding from the accessory arteries. For this reason, it is very important to evaluate liver vascularization in detail during hepatic angiography and to perform arterial mapping studies.

Angiography begins with the entering to femoral arteria and the evaluation of all abdominal vessels that are likely to feed the liver. Thus, arterial vascularization of the liver is revealed in detail. Then, it is planned where the treatment is to be performed by entering the arteries feeding the lobe, segment, or subsegmentary part.

At this stage, embolization with coil of gastroduodenal, right gastric artery, and some accessory arteries is preferred in order to prevent some treatment-related complications such as radiomicroshpere leakage and gastroduodenal ulcer. After each procedure, contrast is given to test the success of the coil embolization and make sure that whether there is contrast transmission to the gastrointestinal tract or lungs or not.

Hepatic artery perfusion scintigraphy: After the detection of artery feeding the lob, segment or the area constituted by the segments where the treatment wanted to applied and coil-embolization to accessory vessels to prevent possible leakage to the gastrointestinal area during hepatic angiography 5 cc volume of Tc99m-macrogrege albumin (MAA) are intra-arterially injected. After this procedure, it is necessary to monitor the patient in the nuclear medicine department within 1 hour.

Hepatic artery perfusion scintigraphy is performed both to predict the distribution of Y-90 microspheres, which will be applied in the same way for the same treatment, and to detect possible radioactivity escape to the gastrointestinal tract and lung by imaging the distribution of radioactivity in the liver. As the imaging technique, thoracic or abdominal planar imaging and abdominal spot planar imaging with thoracic and abdominal computed tomography and additionally single photon emission tomography (SPECT) or SPECT/CT hybrid cross-sectional imaging methods are preferred (**Figure 1**).

The received images are evaluated visually, and the gastrointestinal system is checked for radioactivity leakage. Regardless of the amount and location in the presence of a leakage to the gastrointestinal system, the patient is considered as contraindicated to the treatment. In this case, the patient is subjected to another hepatic angiography again, and an accessory vein

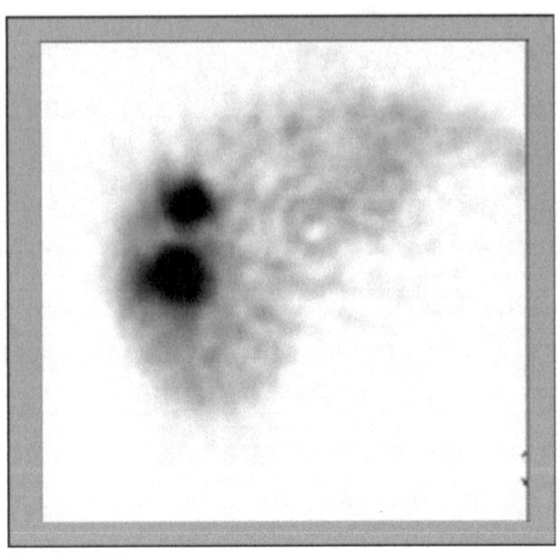

Figure 1. Abdominal spot planar imaging is performed to predict the distribution of Y-90 microspheres, which will be applied in the same way for the treatment and to detect possible radioactivity escape to the gastrointestinal tract in this patient.

which has caused the erosion and has not undergone coiling-embolization in the previous study is investigated and coil embolization applied to prevent leakage. Y-90 microsphere treatment is discontinued if it is determined by the interventional radiologist that coiling-embolization of all possible accessory arteries in the patient has been made and that there is no other artery to cause erosion.

Semiquantitative assessment is also performed with visual evaluation in hepatic artery perfusion scintigraphy. The aim of semiquantitative assessment is to quantitatively determine the possible radioactivity shunt ratio (hepatopulmonary shunt) from the liver to bilateral lungs. For this, region of interest (ROI) is drawn on images taken from the anterior and posterior projections of the liver and bilateral lungs in torso or half-body imaging. Pulmonary shunt ratio is calculated using the below formula [3, 4]:

$$\text{Pulmonary shunt ratio } (\%) = \frac{\text{Geometric mean of lung counts (anterior and posterior)} \times 100}{\text{Geometric mean of lung + liver counts (anterior and posterior)}} \quad (1)$$

When the rate of lung shunt is 20% or more in resinous Y-90 microsphere therapy is a contraindication to treatment. If shunt ratio is between 10 and 20%, it is recommended to reduce the dose as shown below, whereas the shunt ratio is less than 10%, indicating that the calculated dose can be given to the patient. If the shunt ratio is less than 10%, it is suggested that all of the calculated dose can be given to the patient. If the shunt rate is between 10 and 20%, it is recommended to reduce the dose as shown below for the treatment [3] (**Table 2**).

SPECT/CT imaging is more successful than SPECT/CT hybrid planar imaging and only SPECT imaging in determining gastrointestinal arteriovenous shunts in hepatic artery perfusion scintigraphy. It is possible to perform a full anatomic localization of nonhepatic involvement in the gastrointestinal tract with the CT component of SPECT/CT hybrid imaging. Another benefit of SPECT/CT hybrid imaging is the ability to anatomically assessment of intrahepatic Y-90 microsphere distribution. For this reason, it is advisable to add SPECT/CT hybrid imaging if possible in hepatic artery perfusion scintigraphy.

Lung shunt ratio	Suggested treatment dose decrement percentage
<10%	It does not need to be done
10–15%	20
15–20%	40

Table 2. Suggested treatment dose decrement dose percentages depend on lung shunt ratio in resin Y-90 microsphere treatment.

3. Determination of treatment dose

When the patient considered appropriate to the treatment in intra-arterial Y-90 microsphere treatment, transited to the determination of appropriate treatment dose. There are different methods which differ according to the type of radiomicrosphere used for treatment.

For Y-90 glass microspheres: Basically, it is assumed that the glass microspheres are homogeneously distributed in the liver, and therefore a dose calculation formula that takes into account liver volume is recommended. Although the target dose for the tumor is not known in this calculation method, it is aimed to calculate the activity to give 100–120 Gy radiation to the tumor to reduce the risk of hepatic fibrosis least.

For the Y-90 glass microspheres, the recommended formula for determining the desire for treatment is as follows:

$$\text{Activity (GBq)} = \frac{\text{Dose (Gy)} \times \text{liver mass (kg)}}{50} \tag{2}$$

A practical method based on liver lobe volume and hepatopulmonary shunt ratio and simple internal dosimetric approach is widely used in routine practices for the determination of the dose of treatment in Y-90 glass microspheres. By using software developed to facilitate the calculation of treatment dose, treatment dose practically can be calculated by using the hepatopulmonary shunt ratio obtained from liver lobe volume and hepatic artery perfusion scintigraphy and the radiation dose to be given to the tissue is estimated to be 120 Gy [4].

For Y-90 resin microspheres: Since it is assumed that the resinous radiomicrospheres are heterogeneously distributed in the liver, the determination of the treatment dose to the patient is performed by a series of calculations based on "body surface area" and "partition model" methods.

Calculation based on the body surface area is a relatively simple and fast method of calculation compared to other methods and is based on the body surface area calculated from the patient's height and body weight and the tumor's volume invasion rate (tumor/liver ratio):

$$\text{Activity (GBq)} = \frac{[\text{Body surface area (m}^2) - 0.2\,] + \text{tumor volume}}{\text{Tumor volume} + \text{liver volume}} \tag{3}$$

The liver and tumor volumes included in this formula are calculated from CT, MRI, or SPECT/CT images of the patient who have been assessed for eligibility for treatment.

In the Y-90 resin microsphere treatment calculation method based on the body surface area, it is suggested to reduce the calculated dose by 10–20% in patients with borderline liver function [1].

In addition, it is recommended to perform the necessary dose reductions according to the hepatopulmonary shunt rate [3].

The goal of the treatment with the partition model is to give the lowest possible dose to the remaining liver parenchyma while the tumor is being dosed at the maximum intensity of the tumor.

This method is based on the "medical internal radiation dose" (MIRD) theoretical bases and accounts for the tumor and nontumoral liver tissue separately. In the partition model, the Y-90 microsphere treatment dose is calculated as follows:

1. Tumor and nontumor liver volumes are calculated by any of the CT, MRI, or SPECT/CT methods.

2. The activity ratio that tumor and nontumor liver tissue will get is calculated using the Tc 99m-MAA hepatic artery perfusion scintigraphy SPECT or SPECT/BT images:

$$T/N = \frac{(\text{Tumor activity}/\text{tumor mass})}{(\text{Liver activity}/\text{liver mass})} \tag{4}$$

3. The lung (hepatopulmonary) shunt rate is calculated using planar Tc 99m-MAA hepatic artery perfusion scintigraphy.

When these parameters are calculated, treatment dose is calculated according to the partition model for Y-90 resin microspheres using the following formula:

$$A\ (\text{GBq}) = \frac{D\ \text{liver}\ ((T/N \times \text{tumor mass}) + \text{liver mass})}{49,670\ (1 - \text{lung shunt}\ \%\ /100)} \tag{5}$$

where D liver is the nominal dose in Gy for the liver.

When partition model is used, D value should not exceed 80 Gy in nontumor parenchyma in patients with adequate liver reserve and 70 Gy in nontumor liver in cirrhotic patients. The calculated dose is also recommended to be reduced by 40%. The radiation dose to the lungs should not exceed 25 Gy. There is no upper limit for the dose to be given.

The calculated dose is also recommended to be reduced by 40% [2]. The radiation dose to the lungs should not exceed 25 Gy. There is no upper limit for the dose that will be given.

3.1. Treatment administration

A suitably designed "dose applying set" is required based on the type of microsphere in treatment for both resin and glass Y-90 microspheres. Dosage application set varies according to the type of microsphere and includes methacrylate armor, dose vial, catheter connection set, and suitable needles.

For the Y-90 microsphere treatment, the patient-specific prescribed treatment dose emptied to the treatment vial with 5 ml volume injectors that settled into the application set. While glass microspheres are compatible with saline, resin microspheres are compatible with sterile injectable water. Once the dose preparation and vial settlement procedure is complete, the radiation dose is measured and recorded by the radiation physicist in the nuclear medicine department with a dose counter at a distance from the four sides of the methacrylate armor. This record is a practical method of indirectly understanding whether the treatment dose is complete after treatment infusion of the dose is over or not.

In the interventional radiology department, when the patient is interfered with via the femoral artery and the Tc99m-MAA is confirmed by contrast angiography where the catheter is placed, the connection set of the dose vials placed in the treatment set appropriately is connected to the outer end of the angiographic catheter. During Y-90 resin microsphere treatment, slow infusion activity is sent. In order to provide to direct the microspheres to the liver without blockage in the set contrast media and injectable water infusions are performed. For Y-90 glass microsphere application, 20 cc is taken from the saline solution placed in the application set and the microspheres are directed to the catheter liver for about 2 min with slow infusion. After the procedure is finished, the infusion is terminated by washing 2 times with 20 cc saline.

It is of utmost importance that the direction of the entire dose calculated for the efficacy of the treatment is appropriately to the liver. It can be easily understood whether the whole dose is given or not in Y-90 glass microsphere treatment with dose counter which is a component of the application set. On the other hand, it can be determined that whether the whole treatment dose is given or not in Y-90 microsphere applications by measuring the radiation dose at the same distance from four sides of methacrylate treatment set after the treatment. In any case where the infusion should be discontinued during treatment, the activity can be indirectly calculated by radiation physician by measuring the radiation dose with radiation counter and proportioning this with the pretreatment dose. After the procedure, it is recommended that the treatment vial be counted directly in the dose calibrator to determine the actual amount of activity sent to the patient. Since Y-90 is a pure beta emitter radionuclide, very careful study of internal contamination is required especially during application. For this reason, it is recommended that radiopharmacists and/or radiochemists, especially those who provide dose withdrawal and set connection, work with double gloves, not to touch the vial directly with hands, and make the habit of working with control list method not to skip any step in the procedure.

After the procedure, measurements should be made and recorded with a Geiger Müller counter measuring the radiation levels lower than 0.1 mR/hour by the health physician to determine possible radioactivity contaminations of the applicators' hands, room, and waste to be applied.

After administration of the treatment, the catheter connection of the dosing set is separated. The interventional radiologist also applies pubic pressure to the patient to avoid bleeding by drawing the catheter. Once these procedures are completed, it is recommended that radiation measurements be made from the patient's liver area over the skin and at a distance of 1 m.

4. Bremsstrahlung imaging after treatment

Although the saline in treatment application vial can be determined with the measurements during the procedure that the dose is given to the patient by interventional radiologists and nuclear medicine practitioners, the imaging immediately after treatment is of great importance to ensure that the activity is delivered to the desired site in the liver and that there are no undesirable activity leaks in the nonliver tissues.

Since the Y-90 is a pure beta emitter, X-rays that are generated by Bremsstrahlung effect can be displayed under the gamma camera. As well as Bremsstrahlung imaging may be carried out without collimator, if low leveled collimator is settled it may be done in 20% windows that adjusted to 80 keV energy, or if medium-energy collimator is used in 20% windows that adjusted to 159 keV by taking plenary images similar to Tc99m-MAA hepatic artery perfusion scintigraphy, but more preferred method is to take planar images similar to 20% pencil Tc99m-MAA hepatic artery perfusion scintigraphy with 20% pencil adjusted to 80 keV energy or 20% pencil adjusted to average 159 keV if medium-energy collimator is used if low energy collimator is placed. Imaging is recommended within the first 24 hours after treatment [5].

As an alternative to Bremsstrahlung imaging, post-treatment biodistributions of Y-90 microspheres can be displayed by PET/CT imaging in recent years. However, the Y-90 is a pure beta emitter radionuclide, but it also degrades the radioactive decay of the positrons by 1 per 32 million. Based on this characteristic, patients can be monitored directly at the PET/CT unit after treatment. However, in order to obtain a good quality image, it is recommended imaging for at least 30 min per bed position and placing a 2.5-mm thick copper ring in the gantry to prevent the detector from saturation [6].

5. Patient management after treatment

Since Y-90 is a pure beta emitter radionuclide, it is not necessary to take special radiation safety precautions in patients after treatment. After Y-90 microsphere treatment, the patient can be discharged similar to planned angiography procedure after for several hours following time for hemorrhage control. However, since the vast majority of patients are terminal period cancer patients and are likely to have additional internal problems it is suggested that it will be good to hospitalize these patients and the patients are admitted at least 1 day after treatment in most centers.

It is recommended that antipyretic and antiemetic and antiacid medications be given to the patient on the day of treatment against nausea-vomiting and fever which are early side effects of treatment. In patients, the same drugs are continued after treatment and full blood counts and blood biochemical values of the patients are followed. In patients, the same drugs are continued after treatment and full blood counts and blood biochemical values of the patients are followed. Patients can usually be discharged on the day after the treatment without any symptoms or signs, since the primary mechanism of action of the treatment is not embolization but internal radiotherapy, so that almost no cases of post-embolism syndrome like after chemoembolization are observed.

Whole blood counts and blood biochemical control are performed weekly for 1 month from the patients. FDG-PET/CT imaging is performed to determine early treatment response in patients with indications on 4–6th weeks after treatment. On 2–3rd months after the treatment, assessment of treatment response with CT and/or MRI is done.

Side effects and complications: As well as intra-arterial Y-90 microsphere treatment is effective, it is also a safe local treatment method because of its theoretical basis. As a result, side effects and complications are less common than systemic treatments and other similar local treatments. The most common side effects associated with treatment are mostly seen in the acute phase, most of these are self-repairing minor side effects. Serious side effects and complications are rarely observed after treatment, most of which are subacute and chronic effects that arise after the 3rd month [1–5]. Although radiomicrospheres are directed intra-arterially to the tumor veining and emitted radiation to the tumor from the inside via embolization, the main action mechanism of the treatment is not embolism, causing internal radiation damage. For this reason, the embolization syndrome observed in chemoembolization is not an expected side effect of Y-90 microsphere treatment.

However, side effects such as fever, abdominal pain, nausea, and vomiting can be observed in the first hours of treatment because of the systemic endothelial damage response in patients due to intravascular intervention. It is possible to prevent these side effects with premedication with appropriate drugs such as antipyretics, analgesic, and antiacid-antiemetics and maintenance with same drugs in the first week after treatment; however most of these effects are self-limiting and low to moderate in severity.

The most common side effects in patients are anorexia and fatigue. These constitutional effects may take over 4–6 weeks after treatment. These symptoms usually improve without requiring additional treatment, as patients receive regular oral nutrition and hydration at rest and after rest.

Transient increment may occur in liver transaminases beginning in the first 4–6 weeks and continuing for 2–3 months in the majority of patients taking Y-90 microsphere treatment. This increment is mostly low to medium, and is self-limiting. Patients are advised to check their blood biochemical values during the first 4–6 weeks following treatment.

Especially thrombocytopenia can be observed in the blood counts in the first 3 months after Y-90 microsphere treatment. It is believed that this effect arises due to the fact that Y-90 is given localized and it is a radiopharmaceutical with good in-vivo stability, so that it is not directly affected to bone marrow, it is mostly due to not to production of some blood proteins in the liver as a result of the liver damage and transient failure. For this reason, it is recommended that blood counts followed up for the first few months.

Apart from these effects, cholecystitis may arise within the first 4–6 weeks after treatment in Y-90 microsphere treatment. Cholecystitis usually arises due to a radiomicroscopic leak in the bile of the cystic artery, which is an accessory artery, in patients who do not undergo coil embolization. In some patients, leakage may be seen to the bile duct due to reflux caused by vasospasm during the treatment. Cholecystitis due to Y-90 microsphere treatment gives clinical signs of cholecystitis due to other factors and the treatment does not show any difference.

Transient blockage may develop in the intrahepatic bile ducts due to tissue edema, which is often caused by radiation damage due to treatment. In this case, the symptoms and signs such as an increase in biochemical values that show bile functions such as ALP and GGT, and sudden onset and increased jaundice, abdominal swelling, and severe abdominal pain may be observed. In this case, first cholecystectomy metics and biliary function increasing antiedema medical treatments are applied. If the patient does not respond to these medical treatments, a temporary stent may be placed to the bile ducts.

The most serious complication of Y-90 microsphere treatment is "radiation-induced liver disease". Radiation-induced liver disease is a liver failure table characterized by sudden and excessive increases of total bilirubin levels without significant increases of liver transaminases, a sudden decrease in albumin level, and a sudden onset of progressive liver disease with abrupt onset and increased acidity, jaundice. Although its mechanism is not completely known, it is thought to be inflammation due to radiation damage and subsequent fibrosis. In radiation-induced liver disease, the patient is treated with anti-inflammatory, anti-inflammatory, and anti-inflammatory treatments to support liver function. Fulminant hepatitis and related deaths can be observed in patients who do not respond to treatment. In studies, the incidence of radiation-induced liver disease after Y-90 microsphere treatment is reported to be about 3% [7].

Another serious complication of Y-90 microsphere treatment is pulmonary fibrosis. Performing hepatic artery perfusion scintigraphy with Tc99m-MAA before treatment and treatment dose adjustment by calculating hepatopulmonary shunt ratio treatment complications are rarely encountered [3, 4].

6. Y-90 microsphere treatment in primer and metastatic liver tumors

Hepatocellular carcinoma (HCC) is the most common primary liver tumor and is still among the deadliest cancers. The main treatment of HCC is the curative surgery. However, other treatment approaches, including Y-90 microsphere treatment, are on the way to patients in whom surgical treatment is not possible. It is preferable that a council consisting of a gastroenterologist, a surgeon, a medical oncologist, an interventional radiologist, and a nuclear medicine doctor should be established for the decision of treatment of HCC patients.

In the study conducted by Salem et al. with 291 HCC patients, it has been reported that Child-Pugh A patients are the patients who got greatest benefit from Y-90 microsphere treatment and treatment respond did not change for this patient group whether vascular invasion is seen or not [8]. In the same study, it was reported that the patients had the most fatigue side effects with 57% frequency and the third and fourth degree bilirubin toxicity was observed with 19%.

In a study conducted by Inarrairaegui et al. with 72 HHC patients, it has been reported that median survival was 13 months [9]. The treatment respond of the patients with more than five lesions, bilobar disease, and alpha-fetoprotein >52 IU/mL was lower and prognosis of these cases was worse.

Studies have been published the report on the success of the Y-90 microsphere treatment in the case of portal vein thrombosis in HCC patients.

In a study conducted by Kulik et al. who considered the patients with lung and adrenal metastasis HCC contradicted to the treatment, it has been reported that Y-90 microsphere treatment in patients with vascular invasion had a survival of approximately 3 months (10.1 months versus 10.1 months) [10].

Kooby et al. compared the chemoembolization and Y-90 microsphere treatment in their studies. As a result of the study, they have reported that these two treatment methods showed similar progression-free survival rates in HCC patients [11].

Carr et al. compared the patients with advanced phase and inoperable biopsy diagnosed HCC patients in their study conducted in North America. As a result of the study, they have reported that treatment success was similar for both groups [12].

In patients with HCC, a significant decrease in tumor burden is achieved after Y-90 microsphere treatment, and in some patients, the possibility of surgery or transplantation arises and treatment at appropriate centers serves this purpose as well [13].

In addition to HCC, Y-90 microsphere treatment for cholangiocarcinomas from primary liver tumors is performed in eligible patients.

In a meta-analysis study conducted by Al-Adra et al. in a recent year that included a total of 12 studies that examined Y-90 microsphere treatment efficiency, it has been reported that median survival of the patients was 15.5 months, the partial response rate in treatment responses assessed by radiological methods was 28%, and stable disease was reported to be 54% [14]. In the same study, it was emphasized that Y-90 microsphere treatment provided much better survival rates than all other treatments in cholangiocarcinomas.

Serum alpha-fetoprotein levels and radiological imaging methods are preferred in patients with HCC in the follow-up of Y-90 microsphere treatment in primary liver tumors. Riaz et al. reported that a 50% reduction in alpha-fetoprotein levels after treatment is correlated with treatment response [15].

The great majority of liver malignancies are secondary cancers. After the lymph nodes, the liver is the most metastasized organ. Cancers that frequently metastasize to liver are colorectal cancer, pancreatic cancer, breast cancer, and neuroendocrine tumors. However, ocular malignant melanoma may recur with liver metastases even after many years. If there is a possibility of resection in liver metastatic disease, surgical treatment is generally the first choice. However, it is possible to administer Y-90 microsphere treatment independently from histopathology of primer tumor that makes metastasis if the surgical contraindication is met or if compliance criteria are met for patients with liver metastasis that cannot be resected.

In patients with colorectal cancer, Y-90 microspheres can be used in combination with chemotherapy, after chemotherapy, as a rescue treatment in advanced phase disease in the treatment of liver metastases without surgery. Y-90 microsphere treatment combination with chemotherapy strengthens the response to systemic chemotherapy in patients with colorectal cancer that no chance of surgery option [16].

In a study conducted by Van Hazel et al., it was reported that the Y-90 microsphere treatment added to the 5-fluorouracil/leukoplovan chemotherapy protocol at 3rd month significantly increased the quality of life compared to the chemotherapy treated group [17].

There are studies reported that Y-90 microsphere therapy alone or as an effective and safe treatment modality when combined with a radiosensitizing chemotherapy regimen as rescue treatment in chemotherapy refractory metastatic colorectal cancer advanced phase patients [18, 19].

In a study conducted by Kennedy et al. with 208 colorectal cancer patients with liver metastases, it has been reported that there is a decrement in tumor size in 35.5% of the patients, stable respond in 55% of the patients with BT imaging; well metabolic respond is seen in 85% of the patient with the PET imaging method [20].

Although all chemotherapy regimens have been tried, disease burden is reduced with Y-90 microsphere treatment in patients colorectal cancer that have continuing metastatic disease in liver and that have metastases in different regions or not, in this context other treatment modalities such as surgical treatment or radiofrequency ablation treatment are possible [21].

About 60% of patients with breast cancer lose their lives because of liver failure, which is caused by liver metastases. Because of this reason, Y-90 microsphere treatment plays an important alternative therapeutic role in patients who have no chance of surgical treatment of breast cancer with liver metastasis. Coldwell et al. reported that when the decrement of tumor burden in liver metastases in breast cancer provided with Y-90 microsphere treatment and systemic chemotherapy, it has seen that Y-90 microsphere treatment provided a significant increase in median survival (11 months versus 30 months, $p < 0.001$) [22].

Surgical treatment of neuroendocrine tumor liver metastases is still a controversial topic, and alternative local treatment modalities are needed to surgery. It has been emphasized that extensive patient-participated clinical trials and retrospective studies in this regard have shown that Y-90 microsphere treatment of neuroendocrine tumor liver metastases is a well-tolerated, symptomatic healing, and highly effective treatment [23, 24].

In the literature, it has been reported that Y-90 microsphere treatment provides a significant survival advantage in uveal malign melanoma from tumors that frequently metastasize to liver [25].

Y-90 microsphere treatment is considered to be an effective and reliable treatment approach in the treatment of liver metastases in all gastrointestinal cancers, especially in pancreatic cancer, as it is in colorectal cancers [26].

Author details

Umut Elboga

Address all correspondence to: umutelboga@hotmail.com

Department of Nuclear Medicine, Faculty of Medicine, University of Gaziantep, Gaziantep, Turkey

References

[1] Kennedy AS, McNeillie P, Dezarn WA, Nutting C, Sangro B, Wertman D, et al. Treatment parameters and outcome in 680 treatments of internal radiation with resin 90Y-microspheres

for unresectable hepatic tumors. International Journal of Radiation Oncology, Biology, Physics. 2009;**74**(5):1494-500

[2] Sangro B, Bilbao JI, Boan J, Martinez-Cuesta A, Benito A, Rodriguez J, et al. Radioembolization using 90Y-resin microspheres for patients with advanced hepatocellular carcinoma. International Journal of Radiation Oncology, Biology, Physics. 2006;**66**(3): 792-800

[3] Sirtex Medical Training Manual, Training Program Physicians and Institutions. Australia: Sirtex Medical Limited. Available from: http://www.sirtex.com/usa/_data/page/549/TRN-US-0320for20 US1.pdf

[4] TheraSphere Yttrium-90 Glass Microspheres Users Manual. Ottawa, ON, Canada: MDS Nordion. Available from: http://www.nordion.com/therasphere/physicianspackage-insert/package-insert-eu-en.pdf.

[5] Sangro B, Bilbao JI, Iñarrairaegui M, Rodriguez M, Garrastachu P, Martinez-Cuesta A. Treatment of hepatocellular carcinoma by radioembolization using 90Y microspheres. Digestive Diseases. 2009;**27**(2):164-169

[6] Lhommel R, Goffette P, Van den Eynde M, Jamar F, Pauwels S, Bilbao JI, et al. Yttrium-90 TOF PET scan demonstrates high-resolution biodistribution after liver SIRT. European Journal of Nuclear Medicine and Molecular Imaging. 2009;**36**(10):1696

[7] Kuo JC, Tazbirkova A, Allen R, Kosmider S, Gibbs P, Yip D. Serious hepatic complications of selective internal radiation therapy with yttrium-90 microsphere radioembolization for unresectable liver tumors. Asia-Pacific Journal of Clinical Oncology. 2014;**10**(3):266-272

[8] Salem R, Lewandowski RJ, Mulcahy MF, Riaz A, Ryu RK, Ibrahim S, et al. Radioembolization for hepatocellular carcinoma using Yttrium-90 microspheres: A comprehensive report of long-term outcomes. Gastroenterology. 2010;**138**(1):52-64

[9] Inarrairaegui M, Martinez-Cuesta A, Rodriguez M, Bilbao JI, Arbizu J, Benito A, et al. Analysis of prognostic factors after yttrium-90 radioembolization of advanced hepatocellular carcinoma. International Journal of Radiation Oncology, Biology, Physics. 2010;**77**(5):1441-1448

[10] Kulik LM, Carr BI, Mulcahy MF, Lewandowski RJ, Atassi B, Ryu RK, et al. Safety and efficacy of (90)Y radiotherapy for hepatocellular carcinoma with and without portal vein thrombosis. Hepatology. 2007;**47**(1):71-81

[11] Kooby DA, Egnatashvili V, Srinivasan S, Chamsuddin A, Delman KA, Kauh J, et al. Comparison of yttrium-90 radioembolization and transcatheter arterial chemoembolization for the treatment of unresectable hepatocellular carcinoma. Journal of Vascular and Interventional Radiology. 2009;**21**(2):224-230

[12] Carr BI, Kondragunta V, Buch SC, Branch RA. Therapeutic equivalence in survival for hepatic arterial chemoembolization and yttrium 90 microsphere treatments in unresectable hepatocellular carcinoma: A two-cohort study. Cancer. 2010;**116**(5):1305-1314

[13] Kulik LM, Atassi B, van Holsbeeck L, Souman T, Lewandowski RJ, Mulcahy MF, et al. Yttrium-90 microspheres (TheraSphere(R)) treatment of unresectable hepatocellular carcinoma: Downstaging to resection, RFA and bridge to transplantation. Journal of Surgical Oncology. 2006;**94**(7):572-586

[14] Al-Adra DP, Gill RS, Axford SJ, Shi X, Kneteman N, Liau SS. Treatment of unresectable intrahepatic cholangiocarcinoma with yttrium-90 radioembolization: A systematic review and pooled analysis. European Journal of Surgical Oncology. 2015;**41**(1):120-127

[15] Riaz A, Ryu RK, Kulik LM, Mulcahy MF, Lewandowski RJ, Minocha J, et al. Alpha-fetoprotein response after locoregional therapy for hepatocellular carcinoma: Oncologic marker of radiologic response, progression, and survival. Journal of Clinical Oncology. 2009;**27**(34):5734-5742

[16] Salem R, Lewandowski RJ, Atassi B, Gordon SC, Gates VL, Barakat O, et al. Treatment of unresectable hepatocellular carcinoma with use of 90Y microspheres (TheraSphere): Safety, tumor response, and survival. Journal of Vascular and Interventional Radiology. 2005;**16**(12):1627-1639

[17] Van Hazel GA, Pavlakis N, Goldstein D, Olver IN, Tapner MJ, Price D, et al. Treatment of fluorouracil-refractory patients with liver metastases from colorectal cancer by using yttrium-90 resin microspheres plus concomitant systemic irinotecan chemotherapy. Journal of Clinical Oncology. 2009;**27**(25): 4089-4095

[18] Van den Eynde M, Flamen P, El Nakadi I, Liberale G, Delatte P, Larsimont D, et al. Inducing resectability of chemotherapy refractory colorectal liver metastasis by radioembolization with yttrium-90 microspheres. Clinical Nuclear Medicine. 2008;**33**(10):697-699

[19] Kennedy A, Nag S, Salem R, Murthy R, McEwan AJ, Nutting C, et al. Recommendations for radioembolization of hepatic malignancies using yttrium-90 microsphere brachytherapy: A consensus panel report from the radioembolization brachytherapy oncology consortium. International Journal of Radiation Oncology, Biology, Physics. 2007;**68**(1):13-23

[20] Kennedy AS, Coldwell D, Nutting C, Murthy R, Wertman DE Jr, Loehr SP, et al. Resin 90Y-microsphere brachytherapy for unresectable colorectal liver metastases: Modern USA experience. International Journal of Radiation Oncology, Biology, Physics. 2006;**65**(2): 412-425

[21] Hoffmann RT, Jakobs TF, Kubisch CH, Stemmler HJ, Trumm C, Tatsch K, et al. Radiofrequency ablation after selective internal radiation therapy with Yttrium 90 microspheres in metastatic liver disease-Is it feasible? European Journal of Radiology. 2010;**74**(1):199-205

[22] Coldwell DM, Kennedy AS, Nutting CW. Use of yttrium-90 microspheres in the treatment of unresectable hepatic metastases from breast cancer. International Journal of Radiation Oncology, Biology, Physics. 2007;**69**(3):800-804

[23] Bangash AK, Atassi B, Kaklamani V, Rhee TK, Yu M, Lewandowski RJ, et al. 90Y radioembolization of metastatic breast cancer to the liver: Toxicity, imaging response, survival. Journal of Vascular and Interventional Radiology. 2007;**18**(5):621-628

[24] Kalinowski M, Dressler M, König A, El-Sheik M, Rinke A, Höffken H, et al. Selective internal radiotherapy with yttrium-90 microspheres for hepatic metastatic neuroendocrine tumors: A prospective single center study. Digestion. 2009;**79**(3):137-142

[25] Eldredge-Hindy H, Ohri N, Anne PR, Eschelman D, Gonsalves C, Intenzo C, et al. Ytrium-90 microsphere brachytherapy for liver metastases from uveal melanoma: Clinical outcomes and the predictive value of fluorodeoxyglucose positron emission tomography. American Journal of Clinical Oncology. 2016;**39**(2):189-95.

[26] Michl M, Haug AR, Jakobs TF, Paprottka P, Hoffmann RT, Bartenstein P, et al. Radioembolization with yttrium-90 microspheres (SIRT) in pancreatic cancer patients with liver metastases: Efficacy, safety and prognostic factors. Oncology. 2014;**86**(1):24-32